all you need to know about

Heart Attack

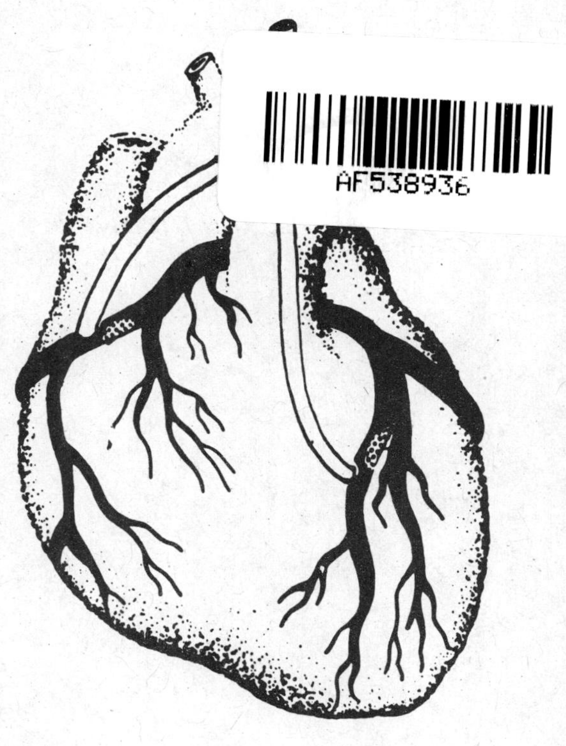

Dedicated to the memory
of
My Parents

All you need to know about

Heart Attack

(4th Revised & Enlarged Edition)

Dr G.D. Thapar, M.D.

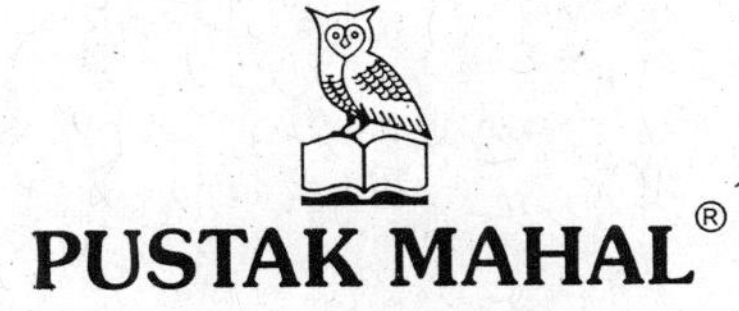

PUSTAK MAHAL®

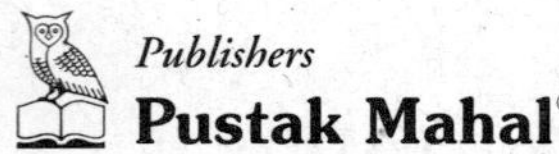

Publishers
Pustak Mahal®

Administrative office and sale centre
J-3/16 , Daryaganj, New Delhi-110002
☎ 23276539, 23272783, 23272784 • *Fax:* 011-23260518
E-mail: info@pustakmahal.com • *Website:* www.pustakmahal.com

Branches
Bengaluru: ☎ 080-22234025 • *Telefax:* 080-22240209
E-mail: pustak@airtelmail.in • pustak@sancharnet.in
Mumbai: ☎ 022-22010941, 022-22053387
E-mail: rapidex@bom5.vsnl.net.in
Patna: ☎ 0612-3294193 • *Telefax:* 0612-2302719
E-mail: rapidexptn@rediffmail.com

ISBN 978-81-223-0011-6

Edition: 2003

Reprint Edition: January 2013

Author's Note
The information contained in this book is intended to supplement your doctor's advice and guidance. It is not meant to replace it.
Do not attempt to make your own diagnosis. Self treatment can be dangerous, especially in the case of serious illness.

Printed at : Param Offsetters, Okhla, New Delhi - 110020

Preface to the Fourth Edition

The book has been thoroughly revised and updated, and a new chapter added.

7, Tribune Colony,
Ambala Cantt-133001,
Haryana, India.
May 2003

G.D. Thapar

Preface to the First Edition

The unprecedented industrialisation and urbanisation of our country after Independence, with consequent changes in the lifestyle of our people leading to enhanced stress and strain, have resulted in a dramatic increase in the number of heart attacks. A more disturbing feature is that the disease is now being increasingly encountered in younger people in their thirties and sometimes even in the twenties, something unknown half a century ago.

The aims and objectives of the book are to acquaint the general public through simple but lucid language what is heart disease, how to recognise it, how it is investigated by doctors, what is to be expected from the investigations, the various medical and surgical treatments available today, how to continue living happily after a heart attack (including the sex life), what to do in case of cardiac arrest, and above all how to prevent heart attacks.

This volume presents a simplified, perhaps over-simplified, account of ischaemic heart disease written primarily for the intelligent layman who likes to be well informed on matters of health, and at the same time, cannot be overburdened with unnecessary theories and contradictions.

General practitioners will also find this book useful for educating their patients.

My grateful thanks are due to my wife, Krishna, who first gave me the idea to write this book and Air Vice Marshal R.K. Mehra for carefully going through the manuscript and making several useful suggestions.

G.D. Thapar

Contents

1

Introduction

Life is immortal, but we all are mortal. On the face of it, the two parts of the above statement appear to be contradictory, but they are not, as attested to by the following facts.

The unit of life is a cell, and the individual human being is made up of millions of cells. These millions of cells arise from a single cell called the 'ovum' (egg) present in the mother, which is fertilized by a 'spermatozoon' from the father. During the remarkable process of procreation, both unite to become one cell, the fertilized ovum, which divides and redivides into millions of cells which form various tissues and organs. We human beings are, therefore, derived form a single cell belonging to our parents and are, in effect, a part of them. Our parents, in turn, were part of their parents, and so on and the process has continued for thousands of years. All our ancestors are still living through us and we shall be living through our children and their children.

Scientific proof of an indefinitely long span of life, if not immortality, is provided by tissue culture, which is the culture of living cells. These cells can be kept alive almost indefinitely provided nutrients, water and oxygen are constantly provided to them.

What then is the immediate cause of death?

If cells are deprived of the essential nutrients, water or oxygen, they die. Oxygen deprivation, even for a short period, can prove fatal.

In a living organism the essential nutrients and oxygen reach every cell of our bodies through the blood, which is pumped into the arteries throughout the body by the heart every moment of our lives. If for some reason this life-giving blood does not reach a tissue or organ, that tissue or organ dies. If heart stops its pumping action, the whole body is deprived of blood which causes death of the body in a few minutes due to lack of oxygen. If an artery supplying blood to a particular organ becomes obstructed, the blood cannot pass through it and the organ dies. One would, therefore, appreciate why the beating of the heart uninterruptedly and the unhampered flow of blood in the arteries are so crucial to life.

Why do You Need to Know about Angina and Heart Attacks?

The most important and the most prevalent of all heart diseases is the 'ischaemic heart disease', which causes angina and heart attacks, This disease results due to the obstruction by fatty deposits (cholesterol) in the arteries of the heart with consequent insufficiency of blood supply to the organ.

The ischaemic heart disease normally afflicts one during the later years of life. Almost one person out of five above the age of fifty is liable to suffer form this disease at one time or the other. It can occur at a younger age too; for instance, during the thirties and forties, when males are more prone to it than famales. Above the age of fifty, the sex difference gradually levels off.

In the western countries, where most of the previously fatal infectious diseases have, by and large, been successfully conquered, the most important single cause of death is the cardiovascular disease, accounting for almost 50 per cent of all deaths. Another 25 per cent deaths are accounted for by cancer and a similar number by strokes. Another scourge in the form of AIDS has at present assumed menacing proportions. However, these statistics need not frighten you. When almost all other causes of death have been identified and prevented, these diseases generally tend to become the final events of one's life. These final events usually occur in old age, but when these diseases occur in young age, they cause a great deal of suffering and misery to the patients and their families.

You would like to ask a very natural question. Why does a layman need to know about heart disease which is logically the concern of the physicians?

A simple analogy will explain why it is as much a layman's concern as a physician's. You drive your car almost every day. Merely driving is not good enough. Factors such as how to drive it properly, how to prevent accidents, how to prevent premature deterioration of the body work and engine are all important. If a defect arises, it is your job to take the car to the mechanic in good time before further damage is done. It is of course, the mechanic's job to set the defect right, but it is your job to recognize that a defect has arisen. Unless you do so, how will you decide to take the car to the mechanic? Similarly for your body. Symptoms of heart attack do not always appear alarming enough to seek urgent medical help, yet, it is important to recognize this phenomenon as an extreme medical emergency. It is the individual who can feel if anything is wrong with himself or herself and take positive steps by immediately consulting the doctor.

You must also know how to prevent heart attacks, what to do in case an attack has affected someone in the family or a friend, and most importantly, if cardiac arrest has taken place.

You should also know why doctors are compelled to resort to complicated and time consuming investigations for the treatment of heart disease; and what medial and surgical techniques are currently available to treat the disease. The next phase pertains to existence after a heart attack and what adjustments in the life style have to be made for a trouble-free life.

These are some of the reasons why you should read the following pages carefully, understand the contents of this book, reassess your life style in the light of the facts you will come across, and make any changes that may be considered necessary to achieve a healthy, problem-free life.

2

The Scenario

It was a cold Sunday morning. The sky had cleared after many cloudy, rainy days. The sun was shining brightly and radiating welcome warmth. The successful executive felt exhilarated. It was an enjoyable, carefree holiday after the gruelling 12-hours-a-day schedule of work in the office. He took his breakfast, heavier than usual, and burped with satisfaction. He thought he would spend a couple of hours with his friend who lived a mile away on the nearby hill. After he had gone half the way up the hill, he started feeling odd sensations in the chest. 'My chest feels heavy in the middle', he said to himself, 'something is squeezing it'. The painful sensation was in the front of the chest and was radiating to the left shoulder and down the left arm. He felt very anxious and sat down on a nearby boulder. In about ten minutes, the pain passed off and he felt well enough to resume his walking, but decided to return home. 'Never in my fifty years have I had a pain like this', he told his wife, 'but I feel fine now'. She insisted that he consult his doctor, The doctor, after an examination, declared that he had heart pain—angina pectoris, and prescribed the necessary treatment and precautions, and suggested further investigations.

The executive hardly paid any attention to his doctor's advice. Angina would afflict him on and off. One day he woke up at about three in the morning with the same pain constricting the front of his chest. The pain was radiating to the left shoulder and arm. He thought it was the same angina and would soon settle down. Only now the pain was more severe. He put a tablet of nitroglycerine, which had been prescribed to him, under his tongue. No effect. He took a second one and a third, but the pain would not relent. It went on waxing and waning. Cold sweat was now gathering on his forehead, and his whole body was drenched in sweat as if bathed in cold water. He felt so weak that even lifting a finger required a great effort. Soon he found his breathing had become difficult. He was now alarmed. The doctor was called in. His verdict: Myocardial infarction—acute heart attack. His advice: immediate admission to the hospital intensive coronary care unit.

3

The Heart and the Blood Vessels

In this chapter we shall take up some basic facts about the structure and functions of the heart and blood vessels in the form of questions and answers.

Doctor, I do want to know about heart attacks, but why should I need to know the structure and functions of the heart first?

For an intelligent grasp of the subject some basic knowledge of this organ, namely, the heart and its functions is not only desirable but essential.

What does the heart do?

The heart acts as a muscular pump. It pumps blood into the lungs for oxygenation and then the oxygenated blood to the whole body.

What are blood vessels?

Blood vessels are tube-like structures, called arteries and veins.

What is their function?

The arteries carry the pure (oxygenated) blood from the heart to various parts of the body, and the veins bring the impure (unoxygenated) blood back to the heart.

Do you mean, doctor, that the blood is constantly circulating throughout the body?

Yes, of course, the blood is constantly circulating all over the body throughout our lives, because every part of our body has to be constantly supplied with nutrients, water and oxygen, which are supplied through the blood.

How is this process of circulation of blood carried out by the heart?

Before I can answer this question, I should tell you about the structure of the heart.

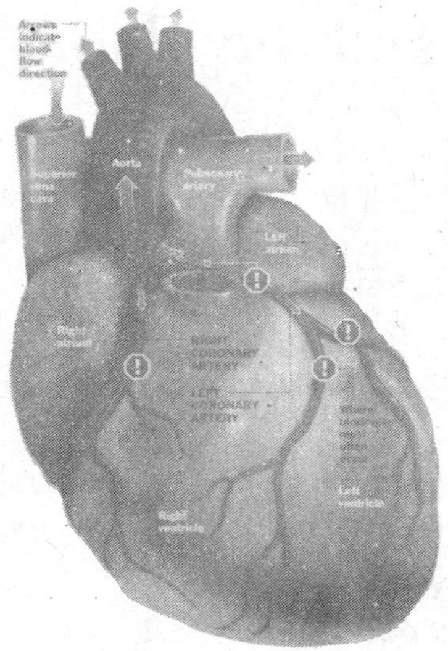

Fig. 1 The heart and the blood vessels

What does the heart look like?

The heart is a muscular structure of the size of the closed fist of the individual's hand, lying in the middle of the chest cavity, more to the left, tucked in between the two lungs. Its appearance is shown in Fig. 1.

What are the different chambers that the heart consists of?

The heart has four chambers, two on the right (actually on the right and front) and two on the left (actually to the left and

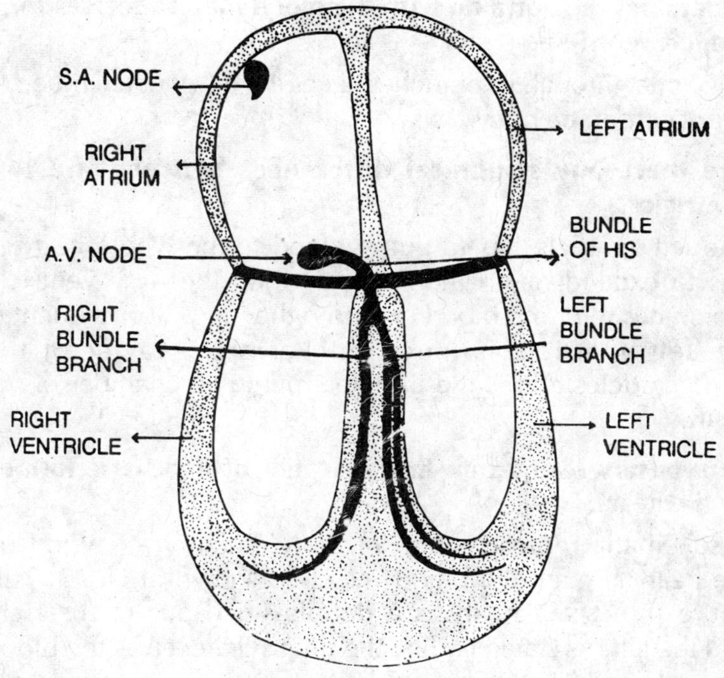

Fig. 2 Diagrammatic view of the heart and its conduction system

behind the right-sided chambers). To make it easily understandable, a simplified diagrammatic view of the heart is given in Fig. 2. Each of the two sides of the heart consists of a smaller receiving chamber called the atrium and a bigger pumping chamber called the ventricle. So, we have a right atrium and a right ventricle, which, respectively, receive blood form the whole body and pump it into the lungs. And we have a left atrium and a left ventricle, which, respectively, receive oxygenated blood form the lungs and pump it into the aorta, the main arterial highway of the body.

What does the aorta do with the blood that it receives form the left ventricle?

The aorta, through its branches, takes the oxygenated blood to every part of the body.

Are there any structural differences between the two ventricles?

The left ventricle has to pump blood to the whole body; it has to expend much more energy than the right ventricle which has to pump blood only into the lungs. Consequently, the left ventricle is much thicker and heavier of the two ventricles and is the principal pumping chamber of the heart.

Can you now tell me how the circulation of blood is performed by the heart?

A schematic representation of the circulation of blood by the heart through the blood vessels is shown in Fig. 3. This figure shows the heart as a double-sided pump, the right and the left. As stated earlier, the right side receives the blood from the whole body and pumps it into the lungs for oxygenation. The left side receives the oxygenated blood from the lungs and pumps it into the aorta, which, through its arterial branches, takes the blood to every part of the body. The arteries are stoutly built tubes made of muscle and elastic tissue. They carry the blood to the head and neck, upper limbs, chest, abdomen, pelvic organs and the lower limbs. As they approach their destination, i.e., the tissues, they divide and subdivide into smaller and smaller branches and finally into capillaries. The latter are the finest of vessels and are spread out into the tissues. The blood is finally collected from the capillaries by the veins and through them is returned to the right side of the heart, thus completing the circle—from the heart to the lungs, back to the heart, on to the tissues, and back to the heart.

How does the blood reach the heart through the veins?

The capillaries are the junction between the arteries and the veins. They enter small veins which join to form larger and

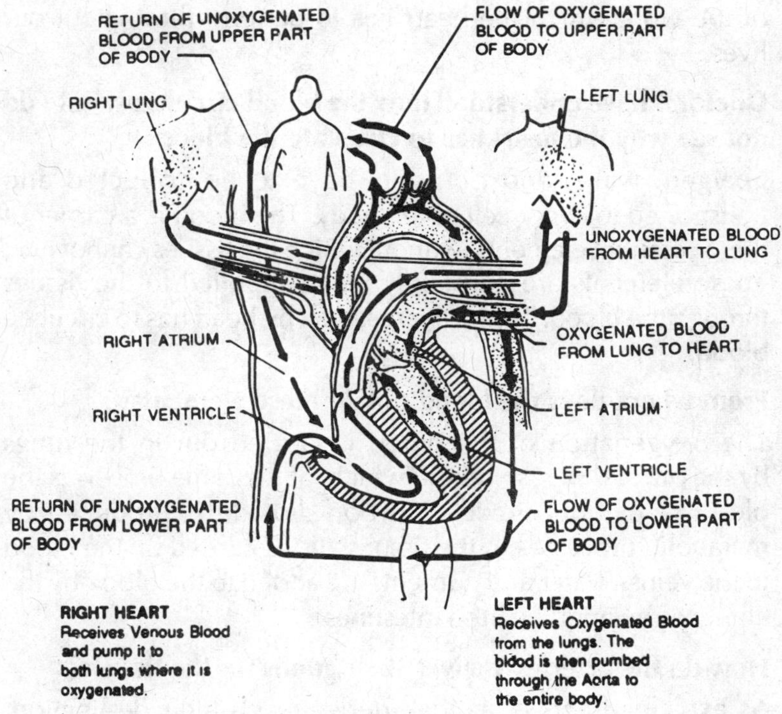

Fig. 3 Circulation of blood through the heat and major vessels

(Adapted form Taber's Cyclopedic Medical Dictionary, 14th edn., with the kind permission of the publishers, F.A. Davis Company, Philadelphia)

larger veins. The pressure of blood in the veins is much lower than that in the arteries, because the only motive force for the flow of blood in the veins is contraction of muscles, in which are embedded the veins. These contractions occur as a result of body movement, acting as a sort of peripheral pump to keep the blood moving towards the heart.

What is the speed of circulation of blood?

The circulation of blood is so rapid that the whole mass of blood (about 5 litres) passes through the body, heart and lungs in less than a minute. You can, therefore, imagine the magnitude of the work which the heart has to perform throughout our lives.

Doctor, I have understood how the blood circulates, but I do not see why the heart has to circulate the blood?

Oxygen, water and nutrients have to be collected and transported to every cell of the body. The blood is a carrier of these essential elements, without which the tissues cannot live. These elements are constantly being supplied to the tissues through the blood. That is the reason why heart has to circulate blood.

From where does the blood obtain these elements?

The oxygenation of the blood is carried out in the lungs by the process of respiration, which, at the same time, rids the blood of carbon dioxide. Carbon dioxide is produced by metabolic processes in the tissues and is carried by the blood in the veins. Water and nutrients are added to the blood by the alimentary canal, i.e., the intestines.

How do the arteries 'deliver their goods' to the tissues?

As explained above, as the arteries reach their destination, i.e., the tissues, they divide and subdivide and finally break up into the finest vessels, namely, the capillaries, which are spread out into the tissues. It is through the capillaries that the plasma (watery part of the blood) bathes every one of the millions of cells of our body. It is here that oxygen, water and nutrients are delivered to the tissues and waste products of metabolism and carbon dioxide are removed form the cells and absorbed into the blood.

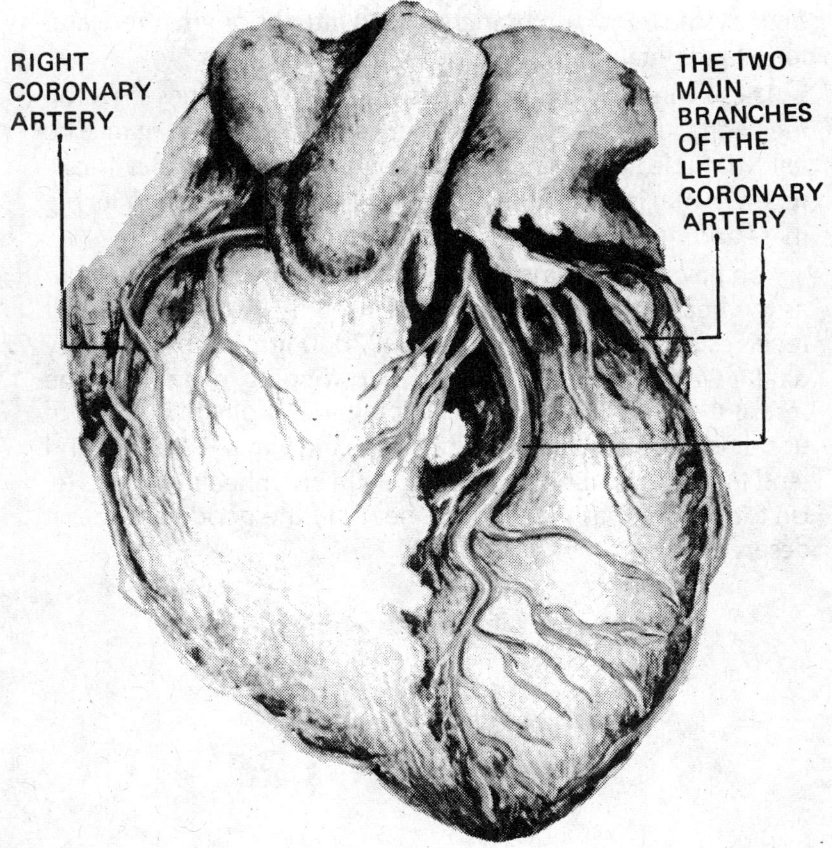

Fig. 4 Coronary arteries

Since the heart has to work so hard, it must be requiring a large supply of blood for its own functioning. Where does this blood come form?

A very important question. While the heart maintains a constant supply of blood to each and every part of the body it definitely needs a large amount for its own functioning. This need is increased when you perform work or exercise. Such a need is met by two arterial channels called the left and right coronary arteries. They arise from the root of the aorta near its origin from the left ventricle (Fig. 4). Since the left coronary artery divides into two main branches soon after its origin, there are, for all practical purposes, three coronary arteries.

These three coronary vessels and their branches envelop the heart, supplying blood to every segment of the organ. The left ventricle, the principal pumping chamber of the heart, receives maximum supply of blood in order to cater to its big mass and meet its large requirements.

You have read in this chapter how such a small-sized organ as the heart, hardly the size of a closed fist, works so hard. It receives and pumps out more than 7000 litres of blood every day! It works round the clock, never stopping, even when the rest of the body is resting or sleeping. It is a pity that many of us do not look after such a vital organ the way we should, and tend to treat it shabbily by indulging in an unhealthy life style. Isn't it proper that we give the heart all the good care that it deserves?

4

The Diseased Heart

Let us now discuss how coronary artery obstruction affects the heart.

What is ischaemic heart disease (IHD)?

Angina and heart attacks are both manifestations of coronary artery obstruction due to fatty (cholesterol) deposits in the wall of the artery, thereby reducing its lumen (cavity) and, consequently, the flow of blood to the corresponding portion of the heart muscle. This reduction in blood supply is called 'ischaemia', and the disease of the heart caused by this condition is called 'ischaemic heart disease' or IHD for short. It is also called coronary artery disease (CAD). Various types of angina and heart attacks (myocardial infarction) are manifestations of IHD.

Figure 5 illustrates a normal unobstructed artery (a), a partially obstructed artery (b), and an almost completely blocked artery (c).

How Does a partially obstructed coronary artery affect the heart?

The amount of blood flowing through a partially blocked

coronary artery will naturally be less than normal, the reduction being proportional to the degree of obstruction. This reduced blood supply may be perfectly adequate for normal functioning of the heart when at rest, but, during exertion, the heart rate and the work load of the heart go up, increasing its oxygen

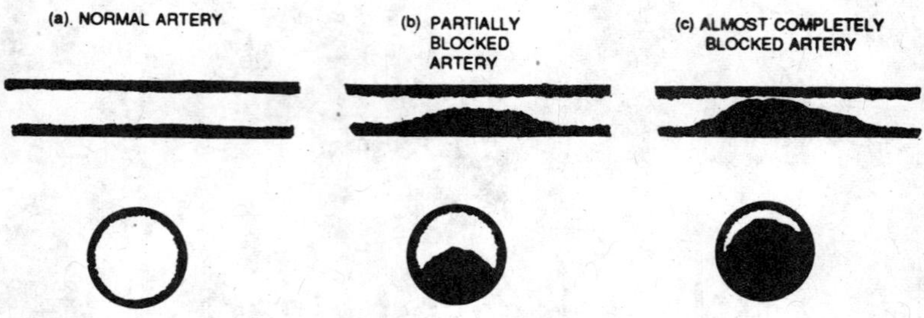

Fig. 5 Normal and blocked arteries

requirement. This requirement has to be met by increased blood supply. Due to the obstruction, the blood supply cannot be augmented beyond a certain limit. This causes lack of oxygen in the heart. The heart muscle cries with pain, which we call angina pectoris or, for short, angina. The pain is relieved if the patient stops exertion bringing down the heart rate and, consequently, its oxygen requirement. When the blood supply matches the oxygen demand of the heart, the pain resulting from angina stops.

Do the attacks of angina cause damage to the heart?

An episode of angina is a temporary imbalance between the supply and demand of oxygen to the heart muscle. The pain lasts for a few minutes, up to a maximum of 20 minutes. It does not cause permanent damage to the heart muscle.

How does complete obstruction developing in a coronary artery affect the heart?

If the obstruction becomes complete, little blood or no blood can flow across the obstruction. The corresponding segment of the heart muscle is acutely and severely deprived of blood and, consequently, of oxygen. This severe ischaemia cannot last long without necrosis and the death of the affected tissue. This is called myocardial infarction or simply heart attack.

What causes the complete obstruction in the coronary artery?

This may be caused by thrombosis (clotting of blood) occurring on the cholesterol deposit, or by spasm of the artery, or both.

Is it correct to say that both angina and heart attack are basically the two sides of the same coin?

Yes, absolutely. As you have seen, the basic cause of both angina and infarction is coronary artery obstruction. It is the same process which causes various manifestations of ischaemic heart disease in varying degrees of severity, depending upon the degree of coronary artery obstruction. There is a wide spectrum of variations, and, therefore, no two cases are exactly alike in severity and seriousness.

Could you please elaborate on the effects of cutting off of the blood supply to the heart?

No living organism can live for any length of time without oxygen, and complete oxygen deprivation is fatal to the affected tissues within a matter of minutes. The oxygen is supplied through the blood along with water and nutrients. If the blood supply to a portion of the heart is completely cut off, that portion becomes markedly ischaemic. If the blood supply is not quickly resumed, the area so affected necroses and dies.

Is there no alternative route of blood supply?

A very important question indeed.

The three coronary arteries are usually considered as end-arteries, i.e., they do not normally communicate with each other through cross connections. Though there are fine (1/10 mm wide) inter-communicating channels, they are normally not open and no blood flows through them. Their number is genetically determined. Under certain conditions, these channels open up and provide collateral source of blood supply to ischaemic areas. See chapter 16.

Does the death of a part of the heart muscle mean the death of the patient?

No, not necessarily. In fact, most of the patients of myocardial infarction recover with a gradual process of repair of the infarcted area extending over many months. The smaller the infarct, the better the chances of good recovery.

Why is myocardial infarction dangerous?

When a severe ischaemic episode occurs, many complications can arise, the most important of which are disturbances in the rhythm of the heart (arrhythmias) which can cause stoppage of the heart action (cardiac arrest); precipitate fall of blood pressure, giving rise to the dangerous condition of cardiogenic shock, and left ventricular failure. Some patients may develop paralysis. Sometimes, rupture of the heart may occur with consequent death.

How do the disturbances in the heart rhythm occur?

Due to acute ischaemia the heart muscle becomes very irritable and can fire off extra beats (extrasystoles) causing irregularity in the rhythm. If the extrasystoles are too frequent, the rhythm may become completely irregular. If they arise from the ventricles, they may lead to the dangerous condition of ventricular tachycardia or fatal condition of ventricular fibrillation. The latter causes cardiac arrest and sudden death.

Other arrhythmias also may occur, for example, the heart action may become too rapid or too slow, so that effective blood circulation cannot be maintained. Various types of heart blocks may appear.

What exactly is a heart block?

You see, each heart beat arises spontaneously in the right atrium, form the SA node. The impulse spreads to both the atria, and from them into the ventricles through a specialised conduction tissue called the AV node and Bundle of His and to its right and left branches. (see Fig. 2). These conduction channels may be involved in the ischaemic process. Complete heart block may develop when no impulse can pass form the atria to the ventricles. The ventricles start contracting on their own at about half the normal rate in an effort to keep the life going. Any of the bundle branches may be similarly affected causing bundle branch blocks.

Do such blocks affect the functioning of the heart?

Proper functioning of the heart depends upon the various chambers contracting according to the proper timing and in unison. This activity is lost to varying degrees depending upon the type of block. The pumping function of the ventricles is, therefore adversely affected. The heart may not be able to maintain blood circulation effectively, if this effect is severe.

How do you identify the arrhythmias and the blocks?

They can be suspected on clinical examination, but for their proper identification ECG (electrocardiogram) is essential. In fact, ECG is the most important tool in this respect.

Why does blood pressure fall during a heart attack?

A segment of the heart muscle is under extreme stress of ischaemia, a part of which may be dead or dying. There may be some arrhythmias or blocks. All these factors interfere with the contractility and pumping action of the heart. The contractions of the heart become weaker, lowering the blood pressure. In some cases, the fall may be profound and precipitate.

What are the dangers of a precipitate fall of blood pressure?

If the blood pressure falls below 80 or 90 mm systolic, effective circulation of blood cannot be maintained. As a result, various organs including the brain and kidneys do not get enough blood for maintaining their life and functions. This dangerous condition is called 'cardiogenic shock'.

What is meant by left ventricular failure?

Left ventricle is the principal pumping chamber of the heart. It pumps blood into the whole body. Unfortunately, this is the one chamber which is most frequently involved in myocardial infarction. If a sufficiently large area of the left ventricle is infarcted, its pumping action is weakened so much that it is unable to pump out the full complement of blood received from the lungs, resulting in a progressively increasing accumulation of backlog of blood in the lungs. As a consequence, the lungs become congested with blood, the watery part of which oozes out as pulmonary oedema. This causes severe difficulty in breathing, and leads to cough and frothy blood-stained watery sputum. If this fluid in the lungs gets infected, intractable pneumonia results.

How is it that a patient of heart attack develops paralysis?

There are two ways in which paralysis can develop. First, the inside surface of the infarcted heart muscle becomes rough. On this rough surface, blood tends to coagulate and form a thrombus. If this thrombus breaks loose, a piece called embolus can travel to the brain through the blood stream, clog an artery there and produce infarction of the brain thus causing paralysis. Secondly, a sudden fall of blood pressure to very low levels can slow down the blood circulation in the blood vessels of the brain to such an extent that the blood may coagulate. This thrombus may cause infarction of the brain with resulting paralysis.

Can any other complication arise in case of a heart attack?

Another common complication is a thrombosis occurring in the leg veins due to enforced rest and lack of movement of the legs. This makes the flow of blood in the leg veins sluggish, leading to thrombus formation.

What harm is caused by the leg vein thrombosis?

The thrombus in the leg vein can break loose and can travel up the veins to the right side of the heart and, from there, into a lung, where it can clog a blood vessel and cause infarction of the lung, resulting in chest pain and coughing up of blood. A sufficiently large embolus can shut off a large part of blood circulation in the lungs with a consequent fatal outcome.

How can it be prevented?

Stagnation of blood in the leg veins is the cause of the clotting. This should be prevented while the patient is confined to bed. The patient should move his legs by alternately flexing and extending them at the knees a few times a day. The muscular action helps movement of blood in the veins and thus prevents stagnation. However, if clotting has already taken place, there should be no movement so as to prevent the blood clot from breaking loose.

5

How to Recognize Angina and Heart Attack

You have already read in the last chapter how cholesterol deposits, which occur in the lumen of the coronary arteries, block these arteries and produce ischaemic heart disease. This disease manifests itself in the form of angina pectoris and heart attacks (myocardial infarction). In this chapter we shall discuss the symptomatology of these conditions, so that you can recognize them and take timely action by consulting your physician or arranging for an urgent admission in a hospital, as the case may be.

Angina Pectoris

What is angina pectoris?

Angina is a heart pain that lasts for short duration (a few minutes). It can be considered cry of the heart muscle due to a temporary imbalance between the demand and supply of oxygen to this muscle.

What is the cause?

As discussed in the previous chapter, it is caused by the partial obstruction of a coronary artery by fatty (cholesterol) deposits, so that the blood supply to a segment of the heart is reduced. the supply may be sufficient during rest, but when the demands of the heart are increased due to exertion, the supply becomes insufficient.

How can one recognize angina?

Angina is recognized by its symptoms, their character, pain radiation, and so on. The pain is constricting, squeezing, or choking, or as if a heavy weight has been placed on the chest. Some patients experience severe burning pain in the pit of the stomach or behind the lower end of the sternum (breast bone) and insist that the pain is due to severe dyspepsia. The pain is usually located in the central portion of the front of the chest in the region of the lower portion of the breast bone. Although the heart lies more to the left, the pain is rarely left-sided. The pain may radiate to the left shoulder and arm, right shoulder and arm or both, to the neck or lower jaw or directly to the back into the area between the two shoulder blades. Sometimes, no pain may be felt in the chest but only in one of the sites of radiation, i.e., shoulder, arm, neck, jaw or even pit of the stomach. The patient may feel very anxious.

What are the precipitating factors?

There is usually no pain when the person is at rest. An exercise like brisk walking, running, going uphill, climbing the stairs or doing physical work precipitates the pain. Even a lesser amount of exertion will precipitate the pain if such exertion is undertaken soon after meals. Emotional outbursts, anger, fright, hurry or sexual activity may induce such pain.

How can this pain be relieved?

It can be relieved by stopping the exertion and by resting. It can be immediately relieved by nitroglycerine (Angised).

How long does this pain last?

It does not last more than a few minutes. However, if it lasts more than 20 minutes, some other cause such as myocardial infarction should be considered. After the pain has been relieved, the patient feels well enough to resume his normal activity. The important point to be noted is that the pain is produced by physical or emotional activity, and is relieved by rest or nitroglycerine, and is short-lived.

Is every anginal pain related to exercise or exertion?

No, there is a more severe form of angina which is called 'unstable angina', in which the character and the location of pain are the same as described above, but it may appear during rest, may last longer than 20 minutes and may be relieved by nitroglycerine. Usually, these cases end up in myocardial infarction.

How can it be confirmed that a patient has angina?

This can be done by your physician by carefully taking a detailed history. Objective evidence is sought with the help of the electrocardiogram. ECG taken at rest, i.e., without exercise, may show some evidence, but, not infrequently it is within normal limits. The patient is then made to perform some exercise and the ECG is repeated to check if any changes of myocardial ischaemia have appeared. (See the next chapter for this study and other special investigations.)

Myocardial Infarction

What is myocardial infarction?

Myocardial infarction or heart attack is a severe heart pain resulting from necrosis and death of a segment of the heart muscle.

What is the cause?

Infarction occurs when an obstruction in a coronary artery becomes complete due to blood clotting on a patch of fatty deposit (atheroma) on the arterial wall, cutting off the blood supply to a part of.the heart muscle.

How does one recognize that an attack of myocardial infarction has occurred?

The character of pain and its radiation are no different from those in angina pectoris, but it is usually more severe, much more prolonged, i.e., it may last for hours and recur for days. Also, there are other symptoms such as profound weakness, profuse cold sweat, palpitations at times, sometimes difficulty in breathing and there may be deathly pallor. However, not all symptoms may be present in a particular patient.

Is the severity of pain a criterion of the severity of the attack?

No, the severity of pain is no criterion of the severity of the illness. Some patients may have little pain or even no pain at all, but only sudden profound weakness with cold sweat and pallor. Any middle aged or older person having these indefinite symptoms will have to be carefully observed and investigated by a physician for possible myocardial infarction.

How can it be confirmed that the patient has had a heart attack?

The physician can confirm the attack by carefully studying the patient's history by physical examination; and by electrocardiogram, along with other laboratory investigations. It is important to emphasize the fact that in the first few hours or even days, when the patient is in a serious state, the electrocardiogram may show no deviation or only a slight deviation from the normal, yet the patient would need all the care given to a seriously ill person. Serial electrocardiograms and certain laboratory investigations are usually necessary to confirm the diagnosis of infarction as well as to watch the progress of the case. (See next chapter for details on diagnostic investigations.)

What are the dangers faced by the patient?

The dangers arise from the complications which have been described in the previous chapter. Briefly, they are as follows:

- Disturbances in the heart rhythm and various types of blocks, causing irregular heart action which may be reflected in an irregular pulse, too fast or too slow, and may end up in cardiac arrest.
- Fall of blood pressure, if precipitate, may cause the dangerous condition of cardiogenic shock.
- Left ventricular failure, causing severe difficulty in breathing, gasping for air, cough and frothy bloodstained sputum.
- Thrombosis (clotting of blood) in the veins of the legs, which may break loose and go into the lungs producing infarction of the lung.
- Paralysis.

It is, of course, not for the layman to diagnose these complications. It is the job of the physician to constantly strive to look for them, prevent their occurrence, and eliminate them through proper treatment when they do arise. They are mentioned here merely for the information of the reader.

Is an attack of Angina dangerous to life?

No, any single attack of angina is usually not dangerous to life, and can and *should* be treated by the patient himself with temporary cessation of all physical activity and by the use of drugs like nitroglycerine, prescribed to him by the doctor.

Patients suffering form unstable angina, however, are liable to end up with myocardial infarction, and naturally, need more intensive and individualised care. The presence of angina of any type is an evidence of the presence of coronary atheroma and ischaemic heart disease, and the increased susceptibility to heart attacks.

It is, therefore, important to recognize the difference between a heart attack and an attack of angina.

Since the character of pain is not different in angina and infarction, how does a patient recognize that a particular episode of pain is a heart attack and not simply angina?

A very important question indeed. The differentiation can be made by observing certain important points: Any heart pain which:

- has not subsided in 20 minutes after rest,
- has not responded to the usual dose of nitroglycerine (Angised) given twice or thrice,
- continues to recur,
- is accompanied by:
  - profound weakness,
  - cold sweat,
  - palpitations or irregular pulse (if you can make out the irregularity), and
  - difficulty in breathing

is likely to be an attack of myocardial infarction and needs urgent cardiological treatment. If there is any doubt, a physician must be immediately consulted in order to decide whether or not such treatment is necessary.

6

Diagnostic Investigations

Diagnosis of ischaemic heart disease is made by the physician by carefully questioning the patient and eliciting detailed information on factors such as the history of his illness; family history; the ages and causes of death of parents, brothers and sisters (if deceased); his eating, smoking and drinking habits; his hobbies, sports and games that he plays; his social life; nature of life at home and at work; and his sex life. A detailed physical examination is carried out, blood for relevant tests taken, urine examined and a routine electrocardiogram taken.

It must be admitted that most of the diagnoses of ischaemic heart disease are made either by a careful study of the patient's history or by the electrocardiogram, aided by other laboratory investigations. Physical examination, i.e., an examination with the hands and the stethoscope, has a relatively minor role to play. Special investigations, like coronary angiography, are done in selected cases.

Doctor, why do I, as a layman, need to know about diagnostic tests?

Patients or their spouses sometimes feel very upset over trivial changes in the blood chemistry or in the electrocardiographic patterns. Savour the following sample questions:

- Doctor, my blood cholesterol level was 200 mg. It has now shot up to 220 mg. Am I in imminent danger of a heart attack?
- My husband went to a party yesterday, and against your advice, he ate an egg. How much harm will it do to him?
- Doctor, you say my ECG is normal. Does this mean that my chest pain is not angina?

You will appreciate the first two questions betray unnecessary alarm, while the third question betrays ignorance, which may lead to inaction. Some familiarity with the diagnostic tests will take the sting out of them, so that unnecessary fears would not crop up in the mind, nor blissful ignorance allowed to delay proper action.

What do we aim to find through these tests?

Diagnostic tests are directed towards finding:

- evidence of a fresh or previous heart attack;
- evidence of reduced blood supply (ischaemia) to the heart,
- disturbances in the heart rhythm;
- assessment of the functional capacity of the heart;
- evidence of coronary artery obstruction and its localisation; and
- liability to develop ischaemic heart disease.

Electrocardiogram

Can we please proceed with the various tests and techniques, starting with the electrocardiogram?

The electrocardiogram is an electrical recording of the action of the heart. It is the most important single tool in the armoury of the physician and is the most widely used investigative technique on heart patients. A typical recording is reproduced in Fig. 6

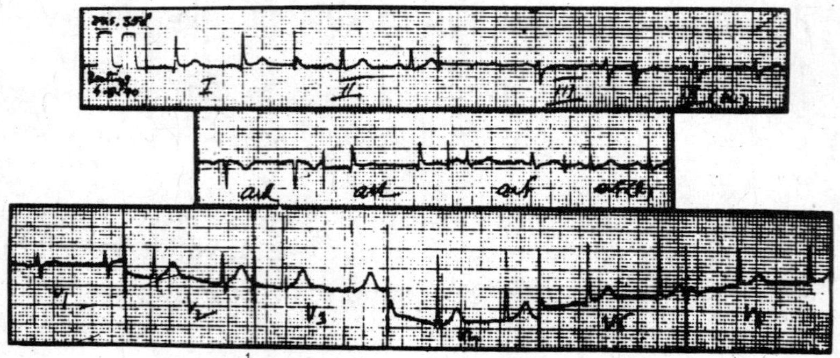

Fig. 6 A typical strip of ECG

How do you record the ECG?

The recording is made by an instrument called the electrocardiograph (see Fig. 7) on a strip of heat-sensitive paper, after the patient's limbs and chest are connected by wires to the instrument.

What are the limitations of the ECG?

In spite of the great importance of the ECG in the diagnosis and management of ischaemic heart disease, it is not the ultimate or foolproof method of investigation. On the basis of a normal ECG, it is not always possible to assert with certainty that the heart is healthy. The ECG has to be read in the light of other clinical findings. In the ultimate analysis, the diagnostic assessment depends upon the clinical competence and experience of the physician, aided and helped by the ECG and other investigations. In the early phase of a heart attack, it is not at all unusual to have a normal or near-normal recording although the patient may be critically ill. And later, after a few hours or days, when unmistakable changes of infarction do develop in the electrocardiogram, the patient may actually be doing better. Similarly, in a case of angina, it is quite common to have a perfectly normal ECG taken when the patient is at rest. Only after sufficient exercise and exertion may changes of ischaemia appear. Conversely, there may be extensive changes of old infarction sustained some years ago, but at the time of the ECG recording the patient may be quite well and cheerful.

Of what use is the ECG with all these limitations?

The ECG gives very valuable information not obtainable by any other means, but no ECG can be read in isolation. The ECG findings have to be correlated with clinical findings of the patient. Only a competent physician with his knowledge and experience can perform this function. Hence, when your ECG or your spouse's ECG is recorded and some change from the normal is detected, do not jump to conclusions, but seek your physician's assessment of the case in the light of his examination and the ECG report rather than the reading of the ECG alone.

What is an ECG monitor?

The monitor is an oscilloscope on which a continuous electrocardiogram appears on a screen. Any abnormality appearing on the screen can be recorded. If an abnormal rhythm appears or the heart action becomes too rapid or too slow, an alarm is sounded. This continuous monitoring of the ECG is done in cases of acute heart attack, particularly when the physician fears the possibility of dangerous disturbances of heart rhythm.

How do you monitor the ECG during normal day-to-day activity?

This is done by a process known as Holter monitoring. A small box-like ECG machine has been developed. It is strapped on to the patient for a 24-hour continuous recording during all the usual activities of the patient such as sitting, reading, walking, working, driving, sleeping, and sexual activity. The entire recording is put through a computer. Any abnormal rhythms or changes in the tracing patterns during various types of activity can then be detected and appropriate corrective action taken.

What are the uses of exercise ECG?

In the case of angina pectoris, an ECG recording, when the patient is at rest, may be perfectly normal. Abnormal but reversible changes may appear only after sufficient exercise

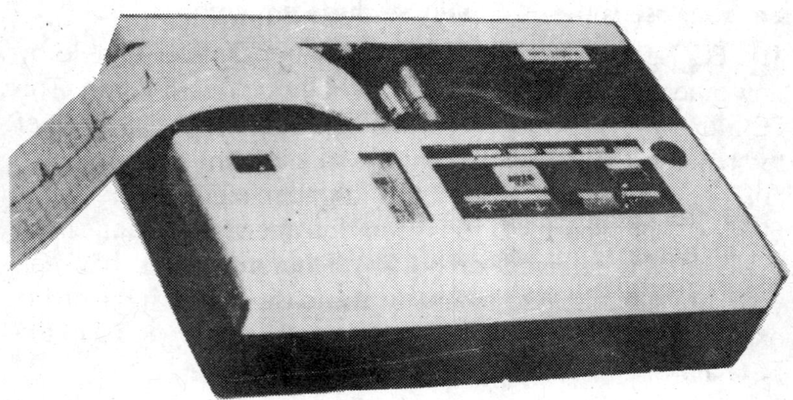

Fig. 7 The electrocardiograph

has been performed. Hence, exercise ECG is used in the diagnosis of angina. During the recovery phase of a heart attack, the physician may want to determine the amount of the exercise the heart is able to accept without strain so that he can advise the patient suitably about his physical activity and the programme of graduated exercise. It also helps the physician to monitor the progress of the patient and to see if his exercise tolerance is satisfactorily increasing.

What are the different methods of recording exercise ECG?

The simplest method in the physician's office is the two-step 'Master's stool' on which the patient climbs two steps up and two steps down repeatedly. The ECG is taken before and after the exercise and the tracings are compared to find any changes appearing after the exercise. The other method is 'bicycle ergometry'. This bicycle is a stationary one, of which only one wheel moves, the resistance of which can be increased or decreased by a system of gears. The work load is measured by the speed and resistance. The third method is the 'treadmill'. The patient stands on a moving platform, where he or she has to make a stationary run as the platform moves at various speeds and inclines. The work load is gradually increased by increasing the speed and the incline of the platform. The ECG changes, if any, appearing on a specific work load, are recorded and studied. The exercise ECG can be very useful in detecting ischaemic changes and abnormal rhythms of the heart appearing during and after exercise and not discoverable when the patient is at rest. Treatment can then be instituted at an early stage. Exercise ECG is also useful in eliciting response to therapy and to the programme of rehabilitation and exercise.

X-Rays

Are X-rays also used in the diagnosis of heart diseases?

Yes, X-rays of the chest are helpful in determining the size of the heart. An enlarged heart shadow indicates an overburdened heart. Signs of failure of heart function (left ventricular failure), which causes difficulty in breathing, may be seen in the lung fields, which become congested, i.e., the lung fields, which are normally translucent, become more opaque. Punctate opacities appear and blood vascular markings become more prominent. Effects of therapy can be measured by comparing successive X-rays.

Clinical Laboratory Tests

What are the various clinical laboratory tests commonly performed on patients suffering form heart diseases?

The most commonly performed tests are:

- Blood lipid (fat) estimation.
- Blood sugar estimation.
- Blood uric acid estimation.
- Cardiac enzyme levels estimation.
- Urinalysis.
- White blood cell count.
- Erythrocyte sedimentation rate estimation.

Fats are generally implicated in the causation of ischaemic heart disease. Please tell me about their presence in the blood.

Two types of lipids (fats) have been implicated in the causation of atheroma (fatty deposits) in the arteries, namely, cholesterol and neutral fats called triglycerides. Cholesterol is the fatty substance that gets deposited on the arterial wall and obstructs the flow of blood. A high intake of cholesterol-containing foods (*eggs, ghee,* butter and organ meats from brain and liver) keeps the blood cholesterol level high and, over the years, it gets deposited on the arterial wall. You will, therefore, appreciate that the adverse effects are the result of prolonged high cholesterol levels in the blood, and just one egg or slight variations of cholesterol levels cannot make any immediate difference to the health of the person, nor can it precipitate a heart attack. The blood cholesterol levels are as follows:

Normal	150-220 mg%
Borderline	220-250 mg%
High	above 250 mg%

There are two types of cholesterol. HDL (high density lipoprotein) cholesterol and LDL (low density lipoprotein) cholesterol. It is the LDL cholesterol which tends to get deposited on the arterial wall, while the HDL cholesterol is protective and beneficial.

HDL cholesterol level: Normal 30-90 mg%

(it should not be less than 25% of total cholesterol level)

The triglycerides (neutral fats) are particularly implicated in the causation of IHD in the Indians. The triglyceride levels are as follows:

Normal	35-150 mg%
Borderline	150-190 mg%
High	above 190 mg %

Why is blood sugar estimation necessary in heart patients?

Diabetic patients are much more vulnerable to heart attacks than the non-diabetics. Many borderline or mild cases remain undetected and the disease continues doing the damage. It is, therefore, important to ensure by blood sugar estimation that no case of diabetes remains undetected. All persons above the age of 50 should have their blood sugar checked at least once a year. The blood sugar levels are as follows:

During fasting:	Normal	80-100 mg%
	Borderline	100-110 mg%
	Abnormal	above-110 mg%
After food:	Normal	upto 130 mg%
	Borderline	130-180 mg%
	Abnormal	above-180 mg%

Has uric acid anything to do with heart attacks?

High uric acid levels in the blood cause gout. It is also known that the incidence of IHD among patients suffering form gout is considerably higher than the gereral population. While the exact cause and effect relationship has not yet been established, on the basis of present medical knowledge, it is advisable to check uric acid levels of all patients of IHD and to take corrective action if these levels are substantially high. The blood uric acid levels are as follows:

Normal	upto	6 mg%
Borderline		8 mg%
Abnormal		above 8 mg%

What about urine examination?

A routine urine examination is done to detect the presence of sugar, protein, pus cells or any other abnormality. Unfortunately, most people get their first morning specimen of urine tested and depend upon this specimen for the detection of sugar, when there is the least possibility of it being found. Blood sugar tends to be lowest in the morning before breakfast, even in diabetics, because the last meal had been taken 10-12 hours earlier. If one has to depend upon urine examination alone for the presence or absence of diabetes, then the specimen collected for test should be $1^1/_2$ to 2 hours after a meal rich in carbohydrates and sugar.

What are the laboratory tests done in the case of an acute heart attack?

White blood cell count: This rises soon after the infarction to 12,000-15,000/cmm (cubic millimetre) (normal count less than 10,000/cmm). It starts receding after 2-3 days.

Erythrocyte sedimentation rate (ESR): The normal rate is below 20 mm in the first hour of the test. It starts rising 2-3 days after infarction and remains raised for 2-3 weeks.

Cardiac enzymes: Injured heart cells of the infarct release many enzymes such as CPK, SGOT, and LDH. Their levels in the blood are measured as evidence of infarction. Since their peak levels occur at different times after the onset of heart attack, they are chosen to be tested as under:

First day (24 hrs) of heart attack	CPK—Normal upto 80 units
2nd & 3rd day	SGOT—Normal upto 40 units
3rd to 6th day	LDH—Normal upto 240 units

Special Investigations

There are some special investigations carried out on heart patients. What are they and what is their significance?

The special investigations are:

- Coronary angiography.
- Echocardiography.
- Cardiac scintiscan.

Coronary Angiography

What is coronary angiography?

Coronary arteries are not opaque to X-rays; hence you cannot see them on an ordinary X-ray film of the heart. If you can somehow inject a contrast medium, say a chemical which is opaque to X-rays, into the coronary arteries, they can be visualised and any blockage identified. Dr. Werner Forsmann made this possible when he experimented on himself in 1929 by inserting a catheter into the vein of his arm and pushing it towards the heart. He was awarded Nobel Prize in 1946 for his work.

What does coronary angiography show?

Through coronary angiography, not only can the coronary arteries be visualised and studied, any blockage identified and their location noted for the benefit of the surgeon who is to carry out bypass surgery but also the left ventricle of the heart can be studied for any defect such as an aneurysm caused by an infarction. This examination is done to determine if any surgery is required and feasible for the removal of or bypassing of the obstruction in the coronary arteries. It can also be used to find out if any defect (aneurysm) of the ventricular wall is present which needs surgical removal.

How safe is the procedure of angiography?

Coronary angiography is an invasive procedure and involves some risk, though, in experienced hands, the risk is small. Since the information it gives is vital for the success of bypass surgery or angioplasty and cannot be obtained by any other means, we have no option but to accept the risk whenever necessary.

How is the procedure carried out?

A special catheter is inserted into the main artery at the elbow or inside of the thigh after anaesthetising the site of entry. The catheter, passing through the aorta, enters the right and left coronary arteries and the angiogram is recorded after injecting the contrast medium (Fig. 8). Thereafter more dye is injected into the left ventricle and the ventriculogram is recorded, which determines the size of the ventricle and adequacy or otherwise of its contraction and the presence or absence of any aneurysm. The catheter is then removed and the point of insertion sealed.

To what use is the information obtained on coronary angiography put to?

If any critical narrowing of the coronary arteries is found in a major vessel, bypass operation is advised. Depending upon the number of obstructions, a one-, two-, or three-vessel bypass surgery may be necessary. If, on ventriculography, a localised

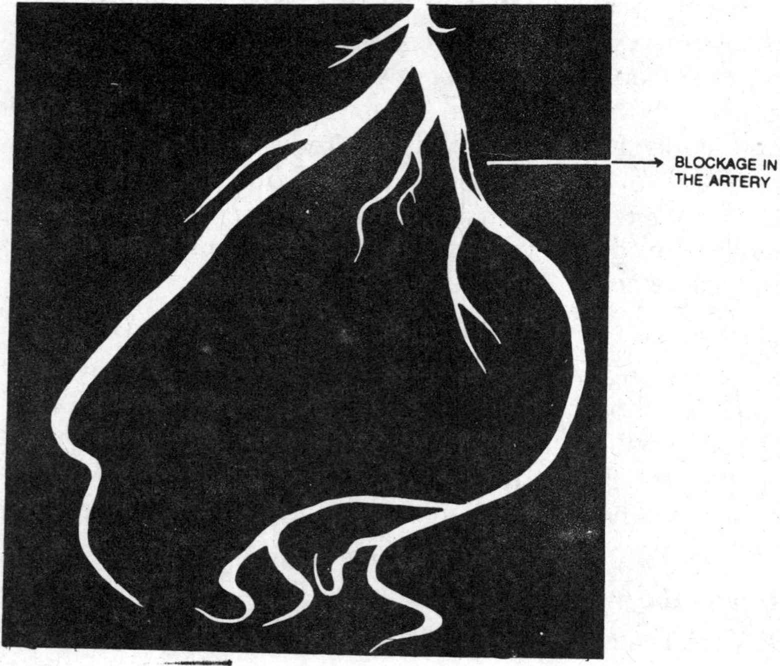

Fig. 8 Coronary angiography

area of disrupted movement of the ventricular wall is observed, it is inferred as scar tissue after an infarction. Softening and thinning of the ventricular wall in the scar tissue may occur causing the aneurysm to form. These changes interfere with normal contraction of the ventricle and its pumping action. Surgical removal of the aneurysm is, therefore, usually advised.

After angiography the patient should decide promptly about going in for surgery. If the delay is too long, repeat angiogram becomes necessary.

When is angiography indicated in patients of angina?

Angiography is advised when coronary bypass surgery or angioplasty is considered necessary in a patient of angina. This happens when angina remains unrelieved in spite of adequate medicinal treatment, or when angina is unstable.

When is angiography advised after a heart attack?

If after a heart attack, there is residual ischaemia, i.e., post-infarctional angina, or exercise testing on treadmill shows high risk of future complications, coronary bypass or angioplasty becomes necessary, and therefore angiography is advised.

If bypass surgery is not considered necessary or if the patient is not prepared to consider surgery at all, should he undergo coronary angiography?

Coronary angiography gives precise information about the location of obstructive lesions in the coronary arteries, which is essential for carrying out surgery or angioplasty. This information does not improve medical treatment. If surgery is not contemplated, there is no point in submitting the patient to the risk and expense of coronary angiography.

Echocardiography

What is an echocardiogram?

Echocardiography or ultrasound cardiography is a safe non-invasive procedure used in cardiology. Ultrasound waves are sound waves of frequencies higher than the range of hearing of the human ear. These waves obey the optical laws of reflection and refraction. They are reflected by very small objects. The patient does not feel the waves as they are directed towards the heart. On reflection, they are converted into electrical impulses which can be seen on an oscilloscope or can be photographed. Thus, various parts of the heart can be examined. The examination can be repeated safely at any time.

Echocardiogram tells us the size of the chambers of the heart, and shape, texture and movements of the heart valves, and function of the heart.

Cardiac Scintiscan

What exactly is a heart scintiscan?

Radioactive tracer material (thallium or pyrophosphate) is injected into a vein of the patient. The thallium accumulates in the healthy areas of the heart, where the blood supply is normal, but neither in the ischaemic areas nor in the infarcted areas, where the blood supply is deficient. Thus, the specific areas can be pinpointed. With pyrophosphate, the opposite happens. This chemical accumulates in the diseased ischaemic or infarcted areas but not in the healthy areas. A sensitive instrument detects the radioactivity, which like the X-rays, is photographed.

What precisely does a scintiscan show?

It shows the actual size of the infarct either by accumulation of the radioactive material, or lack of it, depending upon the method used. It is a safe, non-invasive procedure and can be used on patients who are seriously afflicted with acute myocardial infarction. This procedure shows up the infarct even before characteristic changes appear on the ECG or the blood enzymes.

The scintiscan, being a radioactive procedure, how safe is it?

The exposure of the patient to radioactivity is no more than that to an ordinary X-ray film. It is, therefore, very safe and can be repeated as and when necessary.

What is thallium stress test?

This is a test which is performed along with the treadmill test. Thallium is injected into the blood when the patient reaches maximum level of exercise. The thallium passes through the coronary arteries and enters the heart muscle. Pictures are taken with a special camera and repeated after rest, two or three hours later. Normal amount of thallium both at rest and exercise indicates normal blood flow in the coronary arteries. If thallium is normal at rest but deficient during exercise, block in one or more coronary arteries is inferred. Old infarctions may also be seen as areas where no accumulation of thallium has occurred.

7

Medical Therapy

Medical treatment of ischaemic heart disease has to take two forms: chronic long-term treatment for angina pectoris and intensive emergency treatment for myocardial infarction.

Treatment of Angina Pectoris

What are the objectives of medical treatment of angina?

The medical treatment of angina is directed towards:

- Alleviation and prevention of attacks of angina.
- Increasing exercise tolerance.
- Prevention of myocardial infarction.

How are the attacks of angina treated?

The aim of the treatment is to prevent the attacks from occurring as far as possible and to control the attack if and when it occurs. The sheet-anchor of the treatment is nitrates. The short but quick acting nitrates such as nitroglycerine (Angised) are used to treat the attack. The drug is kept under the tongue, which causes rapid absorption of the drug so that the effects appear within a couple of minutes. The patient should also stop all activity in order to reduce the oxygen demand of the heart. The medium acting nitrates, such as isosorbide dinitrate (sorbitrate), and longer acting nitrates such as mononitrate are used to prevent attacks of angina from recurring. Nitrates are drugs which ought to be given freely. The patient can and should take more than the dose prescribed, if necessary, without hesitation. The only side effect is headache, which is harmless and gradually becomes less and less troublesome.

Other drugs used for the treatment of angina are calcium channel blockers (nifedipine, diltiazem) and betablockers (Atenolol, Inderal).

How do you increase the exercise tolerance?

Nitrates increase the exercise tolerance. Such tolerance should be further increased by gradually increasing the quota of exercise in the form of walking and encouragement to take part in non-competitive games. (See Chapter 10).

How do you prevent infarction?

Aspirin in small doses is given to prevent clotting of blood on the atheroma in the coronary artery. This prevents infarction. Only 50-150 mg daily of soluble aspirin (Colsprin 100) is all that is necessary for this beneficial effect. Larger doses reduce the beneficial effect to the heart and incidence of bleeding complications increases. Aspirin should be taken dissolved or suspended in a glass of water after meals to prevent any irritant effect on the stomach which can cause ulcer of the stomach. Alternatively, take enteric coated aspirin tablet (ASA-50 Ecosprin-75) which does not need to be dissolved in water. Aspirin is not to be taken if there is any history suggestive of ulcer dyspepsia. In that case your physician will prescribe some other suitable drug such as dipyridamole (Persantin).

Cardioprotective drugs such as betablockers are given not only to treat angina and associated hypertension but also to protect the heart from overstrain during physical exertion.

The dose of all the above-mentioned drugs has to be individualised. They must, therefore, be taken strictly in accordance with the advice of your physician.

Treatment of Myocardial Infarction

Why is it important to start the treatment of acute heart attack at the earliest?

The greatest problem faced by every physician in our country in the treatment of heart attacks is the that far too many patients report for treatment after long delays extending over hours and even days. They fail to recognize the seriousness of the problem as early as they should. The first 48 hours of the attack are crucial and the most dangerous and could even prove fatal, for the patient. During this period the chances of dangerous complications occurring are the highest. It is during this period that necrosis of the heart muscle occurs. If treatment were to start early enough this loss of heart muscle can be prevented to a great extent. There are some excellent modes of treatment which are useful only if started within the first four to six hours of the attack. An earliest possible suspicion on the part of the patient or his relatives and the decision to shift him to the hospital immediately cannot be overemphasised.

What is the present-day approach to the treatment of myocardial infarction?

The approach to the treatment of infarction has radically changed during the last two decade or so. Previously, the approach was more symptomatic—treatment of the pain and of other symptoms and then treatment of the complications as they arose. The approach now is to actively try and conserve the heart muscle as much as possible by restricting the damage to the heart muscle to the minimum. This approach reduces the incidence of serious complications and produces a much better end result.

When, in 1982 this author presented, at a meeting of the Indian Medical Association, his preliminary findings on the treatment of patients of myocardial infarction with nitrates and other coronary vasodilator drugs and antiplatelet agents, showing prevention/reversal of ECG changes of infarction, many did not believe them in spite of the documentary evidence; others were shocked that this author was using drugs considered, at that time, contraindicated in the treatment of acute heart attack. This is what usually happens to any revolutionary idea. The new treatment was later published (Thapar, G.D., *Coronary Spasmolysis for Acute heart Attacks,* Arnold Heinemann, New Delhi, 1983) with a report of 19 cases supported by 64 ECG plates to show that the treatment based on the new idea prevented ECG changes of infarction from developing and reversed those that had already developed, proving thereby that it saved the heart muscle from injury and death. The Indian Medical Association accorded recognition to the work by presenting the Best Research Work Award of the year. By now most standard works on medicine and cardiology mention the use of these drugs in the treatment of acute myocardial infarction.

What are the aims of the treatment of infarction?

The aim is not simply to save the patient's life, which, of course, is very important, but also to ensure a good quality of life in case of survival.

What are the objectives of the current treatment aimed at?

First of all, the present-day treatment attempts to relieve the ischaemia as much as possible, increasing the blood supply and, therefore, the oxygen supply, to the severely ischaemic areas of the heart; extra oxygen is administered for the same purpose. Secondly, it attempts to prevent complications as far as possible and treat them as and when they arise, and thus steer the patient clear of the ordeal. However, the physician's job is not over with the saving of the patient's life. The latter has to be physically, mentally and emotionally rehabilitated by gradually and steadily building up his exercise tolerance and making him generally fit to undertake life's future challenges, to do his job properly and enjoy life again as normally as possible, including sexual activity, Unnecessary fears have to be dispelled, not only from the patient's mind but also of the spouse's. The physician has to help the patient modify his life-style into a healthy one so that further heart attacks can be prevented.

What does the actual treatment involve?

During treatment, there are set principles but no set schedule, because no two patients who have suffered heart attacks are alike. They vary in severity and incidence of complications. The treatment must change in accordance with the changing condition of the patient. What may be right one moment may not be so the next; for example, a medication which can and should be given at a blood pressure of say 120/80 may have to be withheld if the pressure falls to say 86/60, and other measures have to be taken to stabilise the blood pressure at a higher level.

The actual treatment is now briefly described. Nitrates and other coronary dilating drugs are given to increase the blood supply to the ischaemic segments of the heart; antiplatelet drugs such as aspirin are given to prevent further thrombosis in the coronary arteries and leg veins. For the same purpose anticoagulant drugs such as heparin are administered. Oxygen is provided to ensure sufficient oxygen concentration in the blood; antiarrhythmic drugs are given to prevent or treat disturbances of the heart rhythm. Suitable treatment is directed towards controlling the fall of blood pressure and prevention of shock or left ventricular failure, if and when these complications arise. Active movement of the legs is encouraged to prevent clotting of blood in the leg veins, even though the patient may otherwise be undergoing complete bed rest. If infections, especially of the lungs, occur, they are treated with antibiotics. Cardiac arrest has to be treated as an extreme emergency by external cardiac massage or by electric cardioversion, if available.

Currently, thrombolytic therapy has gained popularity, in spite of some concomitant dangers and the high cost. In this treatment certain agents (e.g., streptokinase urokinase) are injected into the blood or directly into the affected coronary artery to dissolve the clotted blood, thus opening up the blocked artery and restoring blood supply to the ischaemic segments of the heart muscle. The treatment is likely to be successful if administered within the first four hours or so of the attack, earlier the better.

In many centres abroad, this treatment is followed by angioplasty (see Chapter 8). In some centres, angioplasty is offered as the first line of treatment for myocardial infarction. This approach, however, is debatable. With all the dangers accompanying this procedure, it can hardly be called safe as a first line of treatment for acute myocardial infarction, except perhaps as a desparate measure in desparate cases.

Pacemakers

When is a pacemaker needed?

A pacemaker is required in case of a complete heart block. As you have learnt earlier, heart blocks are of many types; not all cases need treatment with a pacemaker. Some may need a pacemaker temporarily till such time that the block disappears. Permanent pacemakers are required in those cases where complete heart block has become permanent and the patient exhibits symptoms of inadequate blood circulation. The pulse and heart rate remain permanently below 40 per minute. There are other less common indications for permanent pacing, but they are beyond the scope of this book. Of all the cases of myocardial infarction, only a few need a permanent pacemaker.

What does a pacemaker consist of?

A pacemaker is a small, box-like structure containing electric circuitry to fire off impulses at regular intervals and a sensing device which informs the device when to deliver the artificial impulses. The electric power is supplied by a small battery contained inside the gadget.

How long does the battery last?

The modern lithium battery lasts for more than 5 years.

Are there many types of pacemakers?

The earlier pacemakers worked the ventricles continuously. Now, there are demand pacemakers, i.e., if the heart rate falls below the normal rate, they will automatically sense this and send out impulses as long as required. We have now pacemakers which activate not only the ventricles but also the atria, so that they produce a more normal haemodynamic effect.

How is the pacemaker implanted?

A thin wire along with the probe of the pacemaker is introduced into a large vein in the neck through a small incision and pushed towards and into the heart. The pacemaker is then attached to the other end of the wire and is implanted under the skin of the chest or abdomen. It is made of such a lightweight material which does not react with body tissues.

How often should the pacemaker be checked?

Although the modern pacemakers are quite efficient and reliable, it is a good idea if the patient checks his own pulse once or twice a day. If the battery is becoming weak, the pulse will drop by 3-5 beats per minute. The connecting wire may break, so that the pacemaker gets disconnected from the heart. Abnormal symptoms may then appear, e.g., very slow pulse, shortness of breath, dizziness, blackouts or swelling of the feet. If this happens, the patient must immediately report to the doctor who had implanted the pacemaker. He should also report if there is a change of colour, a sign of infection, at the site of the implant, or when the battery starts showing signs of exhaustion.

What is ICD?

Implantable Cardioverter Defibrillator or ICD is a device which automatically senses both fast and slow disturbances of cardiac rhythm and takes action accordingly. It has been found very useful in extending the life of survivors of cardiac arrest after successful resuscitation. These persons are liable to get future attacks of ventricular fibrillation, a fatal disturbance of the heart rhythm. The device immediately senses it, delivers an electric shock and puts the heart back into normal rhythm. On the other hand, if the heart becomes too slow due to complete heart block, it acts as a pacemaker to normalise the heart rhythm.

Are there any other precautions to be taken?

The patient must be careful not to go near radars, electrical transformers, electric arc-welding sets, microwave ovens or any defective electrical gadget. If he do does so, he may suddenly feel numb and dizzy, because the pacemaker's function would have been disturbed. All he has to do is to immediately remove himself from the vicinity of the offending appliance and the pacemaker will start functioning normally.

Life of a large number of patients, whose other organs like brain and kidneys were normal, have had their life-span extended by decades with the help of the pacemakers.

8

Surgical and Interventional Treatment

During the last decade or two, certain surgical and non-surgical procedures have been developed with a view to increasing the blood supply to the ischaemic portions of the heart muscle, either by bypassing the obstruction in the coronary artery (coronary bypass operation) or by removing the obstruction itself (coronary angioplasty). Surgical techniques have also been developed to remove defective sac-like portions of the heart (aneurysm of the heart) formed as a result of a heart attack and which seriously interfere with the normal function of the heart as a pump (aneurysmectomy).

Coronary Bypass Operation

What is a coronary bypass?

This is an operation in which a blood vessel graft is inserted, joining the aorta with the coronary artery beyond the point of obstruction, so that the latter is literally bypassed and the normal flow of blood is restored. The graft is usually made from a vein obtained from the leg, or, more recently, from an artery of the chest wall (internal mammary artery). The bypass technique is shown in Fig. 9.

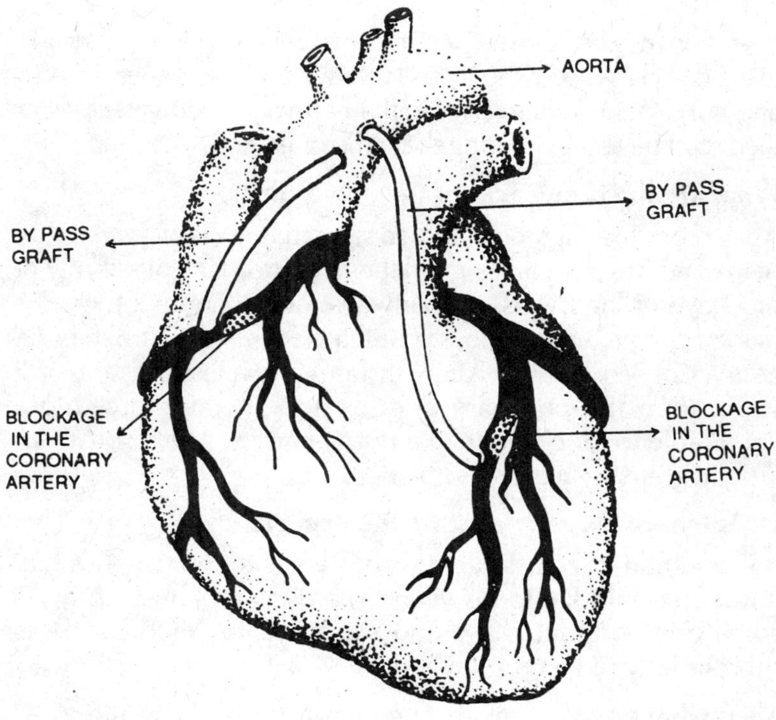

Fig. 9 Bypass operation

How does the surgeon find the obstruction which is to be bypassed?

Coronary angiography (Chapter 6) provides the answer. This investigation is a prerequisite, before surgery can be planned, in order to detect and localise the obstruction(s) and to ascertain if the operation is technically feasible or long-term drug therapy would be more suitable.

Are there any other prerequisites for the operation?

First, the functional capacity of the heart muscle should be adequate. A badly necrosed and scarred heart muscle as a result of previous infarctions cannot be brought back to normality by increased blood supply. However, if there is a localised aneurysm, the removal of which is likely to improve the function of the heart, then aneurysmectomy and bypass operation may be done at the same time. Secondly, the obstruction in the coronary artery should be localised and clearly demarcated and not diffuse. If there is more than one occluded vessel, all of them can be tackled during the same operation.

What are the drawbacks of the operation?

Apart from the high cost and comparative lack of availability of the facilities for carrying out the operation, the possibility of blockage of the bypass graft always looms large. The graft is made from a vein, which is a much weaker structure than an artery. Consequently, it can withstand much less pressure and strain than the coronary arteries and is, therefore, more vulnerable to blockage than a normal artery. The results with arterial grafts may prove to be better.

Does bypass surgery increase life expectancy?

It is doubtful if bypass surgery adds years to the patient's life, but it does add life to his years. The quality of life improves, sometimes dramatically, and the need for medication is substantially reduced.

Then whom do you advise to go in for bypass operation?

Presently the bypass operation is advised in cases where

- the medical treatment fails to adequately relieve the patient of his angina,
- unstable angina which shows no signs of settling down,
- status anginosus which is refractory to treatment and infarction becomes imminent,
- stable angina exists, which is severe enough to interfere with normal daily activities of the patient, and
- critical narrowing of the main trunk of the left coronary artery is visualised on coronary angiography. The chances of survival of these patients are found to be better if operated upon than of those who were not operated upon.

If a patient of angina is well controlled by medical therapy, should bypass surgery be considered for him?

No, the only exception is the demonstration of critical narrowing of the main trunk of the left coronary artery.

If bypass surgery is not considered necessary or if the patient is not willing to consider surgery at all, should he undergo coronary angiography?

Coronary angiography gives precise information which is useful for carrying out surgery. This information does not help improve the medical therapy. If surgery is not contemplated, there is no point in submitting the patient to the risk and expense of angiography.

After angiography, how long can the patient take to decide about going in for surgery?

A. Ideally, the patient should undergo coronary angiography only after he has made up his mind about going in for surgery if he were to be so advised after angiography. In any case he should decide promptly, because if he delays too long, a repeat angiogram becomes necessary.

Coronary Angioplasty

What is coronary angioplasty?

In balloon angioplasty, which is a non-surgical interventional technique, cardiologist inserts a balloon into the affected coronary artery where blood flow is obstructed by fatty deposit of atheroma. When inflated, the balloon expands the inside walls of the artery, compressing the cholesterol-laden fatty plaque blocking the artery. When the ballon is removed, however, the artery can recoil, leaving the opening narrower than it was with the inflated balloon in position, a condition known as restenosis.

How do you prevent restenosis?

The cardiologist inserts a coil, called the stent, into the coronary artery. Stent is a cage like structure usually made of surgical grade stainless steel. It is strong and rigid and becomes permanently incorporated in the wall of the artery and keeps the lumen open by preventing recoiling of the artery.

What are the results?

The initial success rate in experienced hands is about 80 per cent, but about 20 per cent need repeat angioplasty within six months. Without stenting, almost one-third cases relapse within a matter of six months, and the remaining in about four years or so.

Are there any dangers involved?

Yes, about 6 per cent of the patients require emergency bypass surgery because of acute and sudden coronary occlusion causing myocardial infarction and dangerous disturbances of the heart rhythm. Hence, the procedure can be done only in those centres where facilities for emergency bypass surgery are available. Mortality rate is about 1 per cent, if emergency bypass surgery is available, otherwise it is higher.

Aneurysmectomy

What is a ventricular aneurysm?

It is a localised bulge on the wall of the ventricle, formed by a sac-like structure. After a heart attack a segment of the heart muscle becomes dead and, in the course of time, is repaired by scar tissue. Softening and thinning of the ventricular wall in the scar tissue, aided by the pressure of blood inside the ventricle, cause the aneurysm to form.

How does the aneurysm affect the heart?

It interferes with the normal pumping action of the heart, causing congestive heart failure and irregular rhythm of the heart.

How do you treat an aneurysm?

When the aneurysm is large enough to interfere with normal ventricular function, it is best removed surgically. The operation is called 'aneurysmectomy'.

Can aneurysmectomy and bypass operation be done in the same patient?

Yes, in effect the bypass operation will not be of much use if the aneurysm is allowed to remain where it is. Both the operations can and should be done at the same time.

9

What to Do in Case of Cardiac Arrest

A heart attack is a dangerous condition, and the greatest danger is that of the occurrence of cardiac arrest, i.e., sudden stoppage of heart action. If this happens, there is no heart beat and, therefore, no pulse.

Why is cardiac arrest so dangerous?

All supply of blood to the body organs is cut off. No organ can live without oxygen for any length of time, and the first to die is the brain. Within four minutes of such a happening the brain tissue starts dying. Even if the heart starts beating again later on, damage to the brain has been more or less done, depending upon the time the heart had remained at a standstill. In a few minutes, the vital centres fail and the respiration also stops, making the job of resuscitation even more difficult and uncertain.

Then what do you advise?

Under these circumstances, if something has to be done, there are only 3 $^{1}/_{2}$ minutes available in which to revive the heart. In such a short time no doctor can possibly reach the patient. Whosoever is on the spot is the only one who can save him provided he knows exactly what is to be done.

How do I recognise that a cardiac arrest has taken place before I can take any action.

This reminds me of an incident a few years ago. A patient in his mid-forties had a hectic day, and in the evening came, along with his son, to consult me for his angina. I had barely started with the examination, when I noticed that he had suddenly stopped talking and his head had drooped. We managed just in time to hold him from falling down from the stool on which he was sitting. His face had become ashen grey. Neither the pulse could be felt nor the heart beat could be heard. A thump or two on his chest did not revive him. We quickly laid him on the floor. By now he had become blue and had a convulsion like epilepsy. External cardiac massage was started immediately. In a couple of minutes the pulse returned, his face twitched, he gave a cry and opened his eyes. His facial colour also returned to normal. He was confused for a few minutes, then started talking normally. He was lucky that the cardiac arrest did not take place while on the way but occurred in my clinic. However, he was not so lucky two years later.

I taught his son the method of giving external cardiac massage, and told him to practise the same and to teach everyone at home, so that in case of a future contingency it would be useful. But it seems the boy did not understand the seriousness of what had happened.

About two years later an electric short circuit occurred in the patient's house resulting in a fire. With restless energy the patient started putting off the fire, and as a result of the high degree of exertion and excitement, just dropped dead—another cardiac arrest. The members of the family were unprepared for such a happening. Instead of attempting immediate resuscitation they ran to the telephone to call me or any doctor who could come. When two of us arrived it was too late. He was beyond cure. This case illustrates what happens when a cardiac arrest takes place.

What should one do in a case of cardiac arrest?

If a middle-aged person, whether or not he has a known record of heart disease, suddenly shows the above symptoms, think of cardiac arrest; it may be the first indication of a first heart attack without previous warning. Feel for his pulse; if there is none, cardiac arrest is the most likely event that has taken place.

Immediately give a sharp, firm thump with your fist on the front of his chest in the middle. Don't be afraid of injuring the patient—there is no greater injury than cardiac arrest. The heart may start beating again. In that case the pulse would return. If not, repeat the procedure twice. If still the pulse does not return, lay him flat on the floor or on a hard bed and start external cardiac massage as follows (see Fig. 10):

- Lay the patient flat on a hard surface (e.g., floor) with the face up.
- Place the palm of your left hand on the lower part of the breast bone (it is the bone running down the middle of the chest in front; its lower end is just above the pit of the stomach).
- The palm of your left hand should be lying flat on the lower part of the breast bone just above the pit of the stomach.
- Place the heel of the right hand on the heel of your left hand.
- With a sudden firm thrust, press the patient's chest down and then release the pressure.
- Wait for one second (say to yourself one hundred and one; the time spent in saying these words is one second).
- Repeat the procedure of depressing the chest once every second.
- This will make the rate of depressing the chest about 60 per minute. The maximum rate achieved should not be more than 90 per minute.
- Resist the temptation to increase the rate; this defeats the very purpose of the manoeuvre.

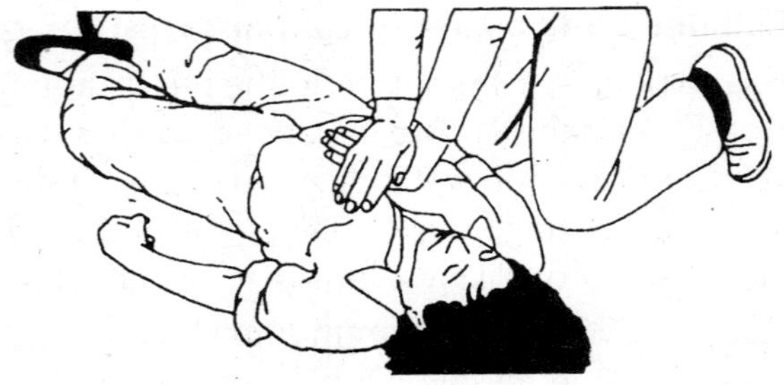

Fig. 10 External cardiac massage

- Above all, be bold and do not panic.
- Continue till you are successful in reviving the patient or till the doctor arrives and takes over.
- If you are successful, the patient's pulse will return, his normal colour will also come back; he may utter a cry, open his eyes and start talking. He may be confused for a few minutes, and then will begin talking normally if no brain damage has occurred; this will happen if you have been able to revive him in less than 3 $^{1}/_{2}$ minutes; after that interval the chances of brain damage and death progressively increase.
- If you find that the patient has stopped breathing, this means that the respiration has also failed and chances of a successful outcome have further receded.

What do I do if the respiration also fails?

In addition to external cardiac massage, give mouth-to-mouth breathing as follows (see Fig. 11):

- Continue the external cardiac massage.
- Extend the patient's neck backwards.
- After every 4 or 5 compressions of the chest, give one breath to the patient.
- Inhale deeply, place your mouth on the mouth of the patient. With his nose closed with your fingers, exhale deeply into his mouth; you will find his chest expanding.
- Repeat the above procedure after every 4 or 5 compressions of cardiac massage.

Not all cardio-respiratory resuscitations are successful; but if you are able to save even one life it is a great job done.

When the doctor arrives, he will take over the case for further treatment of the heart attack. He will also assess if any damage to the vital organs has occurred.

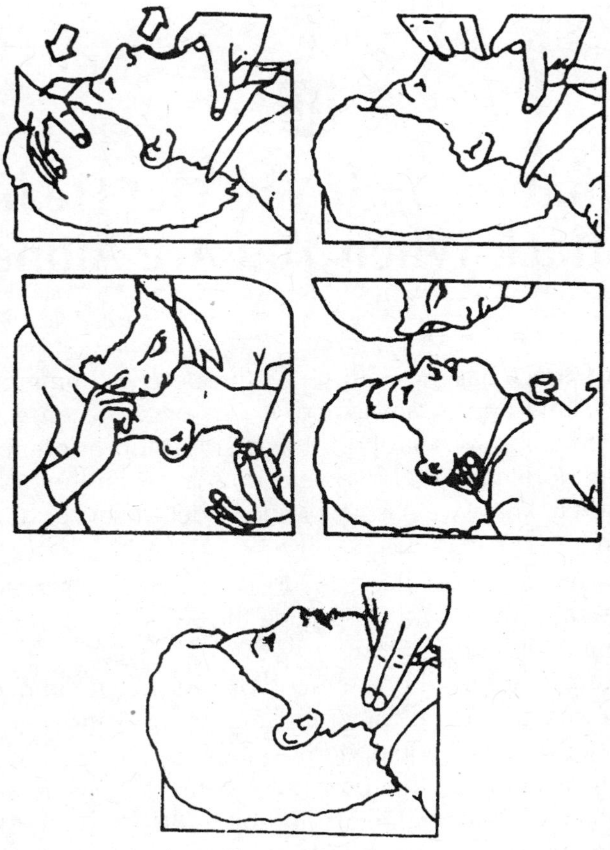

Fig. 11 Mouth-to-mouth breathing

It is important that you carefully learn and practise tne above procedure and teach it everyone around you. Who knows who will need it–it may be you yourself!

10

What to Do if You Get Heart Attack When You Are Alone

Heart attack has the unfortunate property of coming on at any time and at any place. It can occur when you are alone and nobody is around, for example on a lonely road while on morning walk, or while driving a car on the highway. You ought to know what is best to do under the circumstances. Suggestions:

- First and foremost thing to do is to immediately stop all physical activity so as to reduce the workload of the heart to the minimum.
- If alone at home, phone a friend or a relative for immediate help and arranging for ambulance/conveyance for your transfer to a well equipped hospital.
- If driving alone on the road, pull the car to one side, put on the hazard (blinking) lights and blow the horn incessantly till somebody takes note and comes over to help.
- Put a tablet of Angised (nitroglycerine) or Sorbitrate, if available, under the tongue. The tablet dilates the constricted coronary artery, increases the blood supply to the affected portion of the heart and helps lesson the damage to the heart muscle. At the same time, it dilates other blood vessels of the body also, which has the effect of reducing load on the heart.

- Chew a tablet of Aspirin or equivalent such as Anacin, Disprin (not Disprin plus). It reduces the coagulability of the blood by thinning the latter and thus slows down clotting of blood in the affected coronary artery that is causing the heart attack.
- Do not drive to the hospital yourself, if possible. Request someone else to do so.

Cardiac Arrest

This potentially deadly complication can occur during the heart attack or even without previous warning. You may suddenly feel dizzy and about to faint. You have no more than 10 seconds before losing consciousness. The immediate treatment by external cardiac massage, described in chapter 9, can only be carried out by somebody else. If nobdoy trained in the procedure is at hand, you have to help yourself as follows;

- Cough repeatedly and vigorously as below:
- Take a deep breath before you cough.
- Then cough; the cough must be deep and prolonged as when producing and expelling sputum from deep inside the chest,
- Repeat the deep breath and cough every two seconds without let-up till help arrives or the heart is felt to be beating normally again.
- Deep breaths draw more oxygen into the lungs and coughing movements squeeze the heart and keep the blood circulation going. The squeezing pressure on the heart also helps it to regain its normal rhythm.

When you reach the hospital emergency, announce to the staff on duty that you are suffering from a heart attack, making it certain that the emergency has been recognised by them and a specialist doctor has been called in to attend on you. Every minute counts. Earlier the treatment is started, lesser is the damage to the heart muscle, and better are the chances of a good functional recovery.

It is important to err on the side of caution, particularly if the symptoms are not typical such as 'heartburn', 'gas' or pain only in the shoulder or jaw. Insist on proper observation and investigation for a possible heart attack. A stitch in time, saves a life.

11

Prevention of Heart Attacks

Before we discuss the prevention of ischaemic heart disease, we have to know how the disease is produced, what produces it and what factors operate in its causation.

Formation of Atheroma (Fatty Deposit)

You have already learnt that ischaemic heart disease is essentially an obstructive disease of the coronary arteries, which are the lifelines to the heart muscle. This obstruction is caused by fatty deposits, called atheroma, which is composed mainly of cholesterol.

How does cholesterol get deposited in the wall of the arteries?

Blood, which is constantly flowing in the arteries, carries oxygen, nutrients and water. One of the nutrients is cholesterol, which is an essential element for building of certain body tissues. If the level of cholesterol in the blood is high and remains high year after year, such a situation leads to its deposition and clogging of arteries with consequent obstruction to the flow of blood.

From where does cholesterol come?

Like other nutrients, cholesterol is obtained from the food that we eat. It comes from fatty foods, particularly animal fats like ghee, butter, egg yolk, meat, especially the organ meat of the brain and the liver. Our body also manufactures it in accordance with its needs.

Why are high levels of cholesterol produced in the blood?

The common cause is eating far too much animal fats, and not burning them off by doing enough exercise and physical work. However, in some persons the body production of cholesterol is excessive, which raises the blood levels. Saturated fats (those which are solid at room temperature in winter), like ghee & butter, stimulate the body production of cholesterol.

Which arteries are the most affected?

Atheroma occurs in the large and medium sized arteries—aorta, coronary arteries, arteries of the brain, legs and kidneys are the common sites.

The Risk Factors

Atheroma formation with its consequences of heart attacks is the result of an unhealthy life-style in which many factors play their part. These factor are referred to as 'risk factors'.

What are the risk factors involved in the production of atheroma and heart attacks?

They are as follows:

- *Age:* As age advances the susceptibility to heart attacks increases.
- *Sex:* Males are more prone to heart attack, but after the age of 50 the sex difference levels off.
- *Heredity:* Members of certain families are constitutionally more prone to heart attacks.
- High cholesterol and saturated fat diet.
- High blood pressure.
- Diabetes.
- Cigarette smoking.
- Obesity.
- Lack of physical exercise.
- Stress.
- Gout and high uric acid (probable).

You can do nothing about the factors of age, sex and heredity. You cannot help aging; you cannot help being a male if you are one; nor can you choose your parents. All these factors are unmodifiable. But you can certainly modify other factors to your advantage.

I know a hotel-keeper, who is in his mid-fifties. He runs a popular restaurant serving non-vegetarian food, of which he himself is very fond of eating. He starts his work early in the morning and closes late in the night. Whenever I have visited his restaurant, I have found him in his seat with a cigarette in his lips and a glass of whisky by his side, but out of sight of his customers. He has diabetes about which he is hardly bothered. By now he has already suffered two major heart attacks, which have left his heart seriously damaged. Yet he refuses to change his life-style!

I believe you would not like to drive yourself into such a precarious situation. Read the following pages to learn how you can modify the seven modifiable factors to your advantage and stay healthy. If you have already suffered a heart attack, modifying these factors and your life-style becomes doubly important to ward off a second attack.

High Blood Pressure

Hypertension and diabetes are two common conditions which accelerate the production of ischaemic heart disease. The damage is compounded if both the conditions coexist in the same patient.

What is blood pressure?

It is the pressure which blood exerts on the walls of the arteries, and depends on the force of the heart beat and tone of the small arteries. It is expressed in mm of mercury (Hg). The pressure is the highest during contraction of the heart (systolic) and lowest in between the heart beats (diastolic). We express it as, for example, 120 mm Hg systolic and 80 mm Hg diastolic or simply as 120/80.

What is the normal level of blood pressure?

120/80 is generally considered to be optimum level of blood pressure in adults. 140/90 is considered to be the upper limit of normal blood pressure at the age of 40. This figure is somewhat lower for younger and higher for older people.

Does hypertension produce any symptoms by which we can judge its level?

No, high blood pressure produces few symptoms, may be sometimes heaviness of the head. Most people are unaware that they have high blood pressure. It is, therefore, wrong to try to judge the level of blood pressure on the basis of your feelings alone. The correct way is to take a reading with a blood pressure measuring instrument, preferably mercurial.

What are the adverse effects of hypertension?

The high pressure in the arteries causes their degeneration. This high pressure forces the cholesterol into the arterial wall in the form of deposits. Thus atheroma (fatty deposit) formation is facilitated by hypertension. These atheromas, as you have seen earlier, cause obstruction to the flow of blood in the arteries. Occurring in the coronary arteries, they produce angina and heart attacks; in the arteries of the brain they produce stroke and paralysis. Similarly, they can affect other organs, such as the kidneys, eyes and legs.

There is also a direct, adverse, mechanical effect on the heart and brain due to hypertension. The left ventricle, which is the principal pumping chamber of the heart, has to work against high pressure in the arteries. This puts an extra load on the left ventricle, which in course of time enlarges, its function suffers and it may ultimately fail. Acute rise of blood pressure above 200 mm can cause haemorrhage in the brain.

What is the cause of hypertension?

In a very small minority of patients (5-10 per cent), it is caused by other diseases, (for example, kidney disease) but in the vast majority of cases (over 90 per cent) the cause is unknown though theories abound. We call these cases as 'essential hypertension'.

Is there a treatment available which can cure essential hypertension?

No, as yet there is no curative treatment available.

Then, doctor, what do you do to help your patients?

We have effective drugs available for the control of high blood pressure, and normal or near-normal levels of pressure can be produced and maintained in most cases. Since as yet there is no treatment which can radically cure essential hypertension, the control of blood pressure is lifelong, and is imperative if serious complications at a later age are to be prevented.

You will be happy to know that it was an Indian, Dr. Rustom Jal Vakil, who discovered the first drug, Reserpine, from an Indian plant *Rawolfia serpentina,* for the control of hypertension, and introduced it into the modern system of medicine around 50 years ago. Since then many more useful drugs have been introduced.

What are the precautions about salt intake which should be observed by hypertensive patients?

All hypertensives should, by habit, take a low salt diet, say one-third of the average consumption, unless they are being given diuretic drugs. In this connection, it may be appreciated that the greater the quantity of chillies and spices in the food, the greater will be the consumption of salt. If you stop putting the former in your food, your consumption of salt will automatically come down without much effort on your part.

What about exercise?

The hypertensives should perform regular moderate exercise in keeping with their age and capacity. (Details of such exercises follow later in this chapter.) Regular exercise is known to lower blood pressure.

Any other precautions?

The hypertensives should keep themselves calm and composed, follow a regular schedule of meals, work and sleep.

What should one do if the above measures do not bring about a sufficient drop in the blood pressure?

Drug treatment then becomes necessary, which, as stated earlier, is lifelong. There are ups and downs in the levels of blood pressure. Regular checks by your physician are essential for proper adjustments of dose of antihypertensive drugs and to watch for any complications arising from the disease or from the long-term use of drugs.

Hypertension is a silent killer and needs lifelong treatment and control to ward off complications.

Diabetes

Diabetes is a common condition. Like hypertension, it has a long-term damaging effect on the heart and blood vessels, apart from many other adverse effects on the body.

What is diabetes?

Diabetes mellitus, that is its full name, is a condition in which the sugar metabolism of the body is deranged. In normal people the sugar (glucose) is metabolised in the muscles and other tissues with the help of insulin which is secreted by a gland called the pancreas. In diabetes, there is a deficiency of insulin production or blocking of its action, so that the tissues are unable to metabolise the sugar. The latter accumulates in the blood, so that glucose levels of the blood are raised and at these levels (normally above 180 mg per cent), sugar starts leaking into the urine.

How does diabetes affect the heart?

Derangement of sugar metabolism also disturbs the rest of the body metabolism and the blood cholesterol level is raised. This hastens the formation of fatty deposits in the arteries with increased and early susceptibility to heart attacks.

How does diabetes affect the body?

The high levels of sugar in the blood and tissues lead to infections such as boils and carbuncles as well as to diseases such as tuberculosis. Diabetes can adversely affect many other organs, especially the eyes and kidneys. Untreated severe diabetes may cause coma and untimely death.

Can diabetes be cured?

No, diabetes cannot be radically cured with the present stage of knowledge, but it can be well controlled by a proper diet (see section on Food), and, if necessary, by injections of insulin or oral antidiabetic drugs.

Does the control of diabetes prevent complications arising from the disease?

Yes, to a very large extent it does. Many complications such as diabetic coma and infections can be completely prevented. Early onset of ischaemic heart disease may be prevented with proper control of diabetes.

If you are a diabetic, you must maintain proper restrictions on your diet as detailed in the chapter on 'Food' which follows. The control of diabetes is a lifelong process. Half-hearted control measures do not work. The control should be a proper one under the directions of your physician, so as to ensure that serious complications at present and in the later years of your life are prevented.

Smoking

A 28-year-old man came to consult me for chest pain which developed on exertion. He had been diagnosed by a specialist to be suffering from angina pectoris and was taking treatment for the same. The diagnosis, though rather unusual at such a young age, appeared to be correct. His ECG, which he had brought with him showed unmistakable signs of ischaemia. On going through his history in some detail, it transpired that he was smoking 30-40 cigarettes every day. On being advised to stop smoking, he agreed. After one week of abstinence from cigarettes he became free from all adverse symptoms. Even his electrocardiogram taken after strenuous exercise showed no change from the normal. He needed no more drugs for angina. He has become a non-smoker and has remained well since then.

Tobacco as a serious, adverse substance for the heart is now a well-established fact. It is smoked in many different forms — cigarettes, *bidis,* cigars, pipe and *hukka.* In India, tobacco is chewed in *pan* and as *pan masala,* and is also used in the form of snuff. Tobacco is harmful in whatever form it is consumed, though the ill effects may vary somewhat with the form of its consumption.

What are the harmful constituents of cigarette smoke?

Cigarette is composed of tobacco and paper, each contributing to the smoke, which consists mainly of unburnt carbon particles, tar, carbon monoxide and nicotine. Each of these constituents contributes towards the ill effects of smoking.

What are these ill effects?

Unburnt carbon and tar cause chronic bronchitis and cough, which over the years lead to an expanded chest (emphysema) and reduced oxygenation of blood, to which carbon monoxide also contributes. This puts an extra strain on the right side of the heart and can lead to failure of its function (congestive heart failure). Tar and paper are known to cause cancer of the lungs. Nicotine has adverse effects on the heart and contributes to (and aggravates) ischaemic heart disease. It raises the blood pressure, which is an adverse factor for the heart. It causes spasms and constriction of the coronary arteries, thus precipitating and worsening angina.

Cigarette smoking reduces HDL cholesterol level of the blood (see section on Exercise), making the smoker more liable to heart attacks.

Which is the most harmful form of smoking?

Cigarette smoking, because the smoke is inhaled deep into the lungs, its paper content and its easy accessibility.

What is the least harmful form of smoking?

All forms of smoking are harmful, some more, other less. However, pipe smoking is considered to be a lesser evil, provided one does not inhale deep into the lungs as a habit. The reasons are as follows: a pipe is not as readily accessible as a cigarette because it has to be cleaned and prepared; The stem of the pipe has to be held between the teeth, hence a full vacuum cannot be created. The smoke therefore tends to fill the mouth and come out. Cigarette, on the other hand, is held between the lips creating a full vacuum and suction takes the smoke straight into the lungs. This fact is true of *bidis* and *hukka* also. Finally, there is no paper to burn in pipe smoking.

Where do the cigars and *bidis* stand?

Except for the absence of paper, they are as bad as cigarettes.

What about the *hukka*?

Since the *hukka* smoke passes through water, some harmful elements may possibly by filtered out. But in *hukka* smoking also, suction takes the smoke deep into the lungs as in the case of cigarettes and would, therefore, cause the same effects. Since the *hukka* has to be prepared before it can be smoked and it cannot be carried around like *bidis* or cigarettes, it has no easy accessibility. These factors along with the absence of paper make it less harmful than cigarettes.

If a heavy smoker, who has indulged in this habit all his adult life, decides to stop smoking, will it help him?

Yes, certainly. It has been proved that within a year or two the increased susceptibility to heart attacks drops down to near about the same level as that of non-smokers. The severity of chronic bronchitis is reduced and it may even disappear. The high blood pressure falls to lower levels.

Do you advise a heavy smoker to stop smoking altogether or to reduce the number of cigarettes, if he cannot stop it?

It is no use asking a heavy smoker to reduce the number of cigarettes, because after a few days, the urge to resume the original number comes back with a vengeance and may even be exceeded.

Paradoxically, it is easier to give up smoking altogether rather than go on struggling with a reduced number.

If a heavy smoker is unable to stop smoking cigarettes, becomes tense and anxious, what do you advise him?

The second best alternative of a lesser evil, i.e., pipe smoking in moderation without deep inhalation of the smoke. A pipe used this way has been shown to cause less liability to heart attacks.

How to Stop Smoking

Smoking is probably the most important single cause of heart attacks. It is the most significant of all the risk factors, and yet it is removable. Every patient or prospective patient of ischaemic heart disease is strongly advised to quit smoking. Here, I describe a method, which in my experience has been unfailingly successful provided the desire to stop smoking is strong enough.

Does an occasional smoker need to stop smoking?

A healthy occasional smoker faces no problem. Whether he smokes or does not smoke, either way it makes no difference to his health. Of course it is a different matter if he has had an infarction, in which case even a single cigarette cannot be allowed.

Where does the real problem lie?

The real problem of smoking relates to the heavy smoker. It affects his health adversely, and he finds it hard to give up the addiction. His body has tuned itself to live under the effect of high levels of nicotine. It demands nicotine whenever the blood level falls.

We have to understand his difficulties before a method can be found to help him overcome the habit.

How does the heavy smoker tackle everyday problems?

The heavy smoker has, in the course of years, learnt to tackle his everyday problems by resorting to cigarettes. Confronted with a problem, which defies easy solution, he attempts to smoke away his worries and with that the problem. In effect, he has not solved the problem but merely postponed its solution. In course of time, many unsolved problems accumulate. Many a good resolve remains unfulfilled and many a good deed remains undone, because whenever an idea comes to the mind a cigarette is smoked and the action is postponed. A non-smoker would feel anxious about the jobs not done but smoking helps the smoker feel content about not doing the job and yet not feel guilty about it. The resolve of many a smoker to stop smoking is also smoked off by cigarettes day after day. Smoking does not solve problems. It merely postpones their solution.

Does smoking increase concentration?

Many smokers feel that smoking increases their power of concentration. In reality smoking reduces mental performance, except probably when the cigarette is actually being smoked. What the smoker really gets in the bargain is at best a near-normal performance under the direct effect of nicotine, but a reduced performance at other times. Smoking does not increase concentration nor augment mental performance. It merely whips a tired horse.

Why do smokers find it so difficult to stop smoking?

In spite of statutory warnings on every pack of cigarettes that 'smoking is injurious for health' and in spite of the intense propaganda in the press, radio and television about the dangers of smoking (e.g., chronic bronchitis and emphysema, cor pulmonale, ischaemic heart disease, cancer of the lung and peripheral arterial disease), the smokers find it hard to stop the habit. Why?

I am convinced that most, if not all, smokers now understand the dangers of smoking. They also want to get rid of the habit; many have made quite a few unsuccessful attempts to do so. Where do things go wrong? There is no doubt that nicotine addiction is very strong, but why can't their resolve be stronger? How and why does their resolve flounder? The answer to this question is crucial to the success of their resolve.

What are the factors which interfere with the smoker's resolve to stop smoking?

The following factors are worth considering:

(1) The direct effect of smoking on the brain is brought about by nicotine and carbon monoxide. The former is responsible for the pleasurable addictive effects and the latter for lack of oxygen in the brain, which blunts the sharp edge of our mental faculties.

(2) Chronic upper respiratory catarrh with blocked and stuffy nose is a common accompaniment of smoking cigarettes resulting from the irritant effect of tobacco smoke. This causes a heavy head and chronic headache, especially if sinusitis also supervenes. Any chronic ailment reduces our strength, not only physical but also mental and emotional. We become weak in spitit and, therefore, less likely to succeed in our endeavours.

(3) Chronic bronchitis with resulting cough and expectoration similarly interferes with normal cerebration and thought process.

(4) With prolonged cough and expectoration, emphysema occurs; the lungs remain in an expanded position unable to take full complement of air on inspiration. Oxygenation of blood becomes reduced and consequently the brain, along with other organs, suffers from chronic lack of oxygen. Such a brain cannot think and act rationally.

(5) Any other coexisting chronic illness will add to the above problems, reducing the strength to fight the addiction.

These are the usual causes which keep the smoker's mental condition at a low ebb, not allowing him to fulfil his promise to himself of giving up smoking.

How then do I solve the problem of smoking?

The body system becomes so used to the presence of nicotine in the blood that the moment its level in the blood goes down, the body demands more. But there is one very important point to be noted. The lower the level of nicotine in the blood, the lesser is the urge to smoke. A simple observation proves this point. You will find that after you have slept during the night and have not smoked for 10 or 12 hours, the urge to smoke is minimum. You will also find that if due to some illness you have not smoked any cigarette for a few days, the urge to smoke becomes appreciably less. The easiest cigarette to resist, therefore, is the first cigarette of the morning, the second would be more difficult to resist, and third one still more so. This is a point of fundamental importance in our fight against smoking.

How do I utilise the above facts to my full advantage?

This may be done in the following manner:

(1) Any cough, sputum, upper respiratory catarrh, blocked nose or sinusitis should properly be diagnosed and treated by your doctor with suitable antibiotics, steam inhalations, etc.

(2) Any other concurrent illness or infection must also be treated suitably.

(3) Start postponing the smoking of the first cigarette of the day as much as possible, at the same time, reducting the total number of daily cigarettes to half, with the idea of ultimately giving up the habit altogether. You have to be absolutely clear from the start that reduction is merely the first step towards complete abstinence and not merely a permanent reduction because it will not work that way.

(4) Maintain the reduced level of smoking for about a month. By reducing the blood levels of nicotine to half, and keeping it that way you have already reduced the urge to smoke by half; the body is now turned to half the levels of nicotine and its demands have decreased. At the same time, the irritant effect of the smoke on the respiratory

system has also decreased by half. This has further improved your chronic cough and cleared the blocked nose, enhancing your will-power to resist smoking.

(5) After a month, reduce the number of cigarettes to four or five per day. Maintain this level for a month or so. By now you have further improved your health as well as the will power.

(6) Now take the final plung—give up cigarettes completely. Not even one cigarette should be smoked. All ash trays and cigarette lighters should be stacked away from sight, and no cigarettes should be kept in the house. You may face some difficulty in the first few days, but with the passage of time, your confidence in yourself will be steadily built up. You will find it much easier not to smoke at all than struggle with a reduced number of cigarettes.

(7) During the early, non-smoking period you may make use of such items as chewing gum, clove or cardamom as substitutes to smoking and to curb the urge to smoke. But avoid fattening agents such as chocolates, otherwise you will put on weight. As more and more time passes, you will need less and less of these substitutes.

(8) Always remember that the easiest cigarette to resist is the first cigarette of the day.

(9) By not smoking cigarettes, a tremendous amount of energy will be released for useful work. This energy must be utilised to your best advantage, for example, in resolving all your pending problems or by working on any project that you have had in mind for a long time but have been postponing the action. You would be amazed at what you can now achieve. On the contrary, if you do not utilise this energy and channelise it into constructive work, boredom will appear, and boredom may lead you back to smoking.

Use this energy in sports, games or creative work such as writing, painting or developing other hobbies. Keep yourself occupied, but no smoking please.

How do you feel after you have stopped smoking?

After you have refrained from smoking for a few months, you will enjoy 'smooth sailing' and feel easy in body and mind. You will be much happier because your chronic cough and respiratory catarrh would have gradually disappeared; your chronic headache would be gone, and the need for repeated courses of antibiotics would be obviated. You will feel free in your breathing. This will make your brain clear and your thinking precise, bringing about all-round improvement in your performance.

And of course, you will markedly reduce your chances of sustaining a heart attack or getting cancer of the lung. If you were suffering from angina, you will improve greatly, reducing the need for antianginal drugs. If you are hypertensive, your blood pressure will fall, reducing the dose of antihypertensive drugs.

Once off smoking, how do you remain that way?

You have to beware of only one danger. Once you have been a nicotine addict, a distant urge, a longing or desire to smoke may still lurk deep in the mind even after years of abstinence. Normally this should not bother you at all. But the warning to be heeded is: never smoke even a single cigarette, under any circumstances, because then this hidden urge may come into the open and may lead to a relapse of smoking. You may argue with yourself that you would restart with strict moderation. For a confirmed and heavy ex-smoker, it is quite easy to be happy and content with complete abstinence, but a hard struggle to smoke in moderation. So, once you have stopped smoking, no smoking for ever.

Obesity

About ten years ago a prosperous factory owner in his late forties come to consult me for his heart condition. He was suffering from angina and shortness of breath on walking. He had already suffered one minor heart attack. He was very obese, more than 30 kg overweight. A vegetarian, he had been very fond of sweets, *parathas* and other fried food, but had never found time nor the inclination for any physical work or exercise. With a fleet of cars at his disposal he hardly felt the need to walk either for business or pleasure. We discussed the matter and he agreed to modify his diet and to perform regular exercise. In about a year and a half, he shed more than 30 kg of his weight and, in the process, shed his angina too. Breathlessness on exertion also disappeared. He is now nearing 60, but has no serious health problems and is hale and hearty.

Obesity is one of the biggest problems facing the affluent classes in India. It makes a man (or woman) sluggish, worsens the diabetes and high blood pressure, if any of these conditions coexist, and has an adverse effect on the heart.

When do we call a person overweight?

A person whose weight exceeds the maximum of the body weight range as given in the standard height and weight chart (see Appendix 2) is termed overweight.

When do you call him obese?

If he is 10 per cent (or 8 kg or more) overweight.

How does obesity adversely affect the heart?

An obese person has to carry an extra weight of inert fat. It is like carrying around a bag of that much weight during the waking hours. This puts an extra load on the heart, muscles and joints. The person becomes sluggish. This causes the physical activity to further reduce, leading to more obesity. This becomes a vicious circle. The unburnt fats raise the cholesterol levels of the blood, contributing to the production and aggravation of coronary artery disease.

Why do people become obese in the first instance?

Your body weight depends upon what and how much you eat, and how much you burn off by physical work and exercise. If you eat less and work more, you lose weight. Conversely, if you eat more and work less, you become obese. The extra calories are converted by the body into fat. If the percentage of fat in your diet is high, it naturally, leads to fattening.

Do we need to reduce the intake of fats only to prevent or get rid of obesity?

Consuming fats—*ghee,* butter, oils—is of course fattening. But his is not the whole story. Consumption of carbohydrates, e.g., sugar, sweets, rice, *chapatis,* and potatoes, is also important from the point of view of gaining weight, because our diet contains large amounts of these materials. Our body converts unutilised or unspent calories from carbohydrates into fat. The worst offenders in our diet are sweets, sweet dishes, ice creams and fried food like *parathas* and *purees* which contain both carbohydrates and fat and which stimulate the appetite, leading to overeating.

Some people habitually overeat. They do not stop eating till their stomach can accept no more. They are the ones who become obese. Once a person becomes obese, his obesity can be maintained on surprisingly small amounts of food because of the restricted physical activity.

How does one reduce weight?

There are no useful or safe drugs for the purpose. For the obese the only way to shed weight is to eat less and work more. By work I mean physical activity and exercise (see section on Exercise).

What exactly should the diet, that you advise for the purpose, contain?

The diet should contain enough proteins, which are the body building substances, but carbohydrates and fats should be cut down. All fried food and sweets should be banned. Pulses and milk along with some fish and poultry for the non-vegetarians will supply all the proteins necessary. Take fresh vegetables and fruit in plenty, but restrict the intake of very sweet fruit like mangoes and grapes. Take plenty of salads, which are stomach fillers and also supply vitamins and fibre. Take water or buttermilk (*lassi*) before you begin eating, so that the stomach becomes partly full. You will eat less this way. Along with this diet, take a small helping of rice or *chapatis,* which are the main sources of carbohydrates in our diet.

How much loss of weight per month one should aim at?

If you aim to lose 1 - 1½ kg per month, you will encounter no difficulty. But if you are very obese, you should aim at losing 2 kg per month. This way you will shed 10-20 kg in a year's time.

Are crash diets advisable?

Such diets are not easy to practise, and may cause deficiencies of vitamins and minerals. You may feel a great deal of weakness, which may interfere with your work. These diets cannot be maintained for long and obesity returns quickly. It would be better to aim at reasonable monthly targets. Apart from the ease and practicability of such an approach, the great advantage is that by the time you have shed the extra weight you get accustomed to the reduced diet. With slight adjustment, such a diet can be continued indefinitely so that obesity does not reappear.

Would you advise fasting?

Fasting on specified days of the week may be helpful, provided you do not overeat on the day following the fast. Long periods of fasting at a stretch are inadvisable.

The important point to be remembered in the prevention and control of obesity is that 'slow and steady wins the race'.

Exercise

Physical inactivity, lack of exercise and obesity are important factors contributing to an unhealthy life-style which ultimately leads to heart attacks. Let us examine the role of exercise and physical activity in this context.

Is physical exercise good for the heart?

Yes, and we are beginning to understand why. A complex family of particles called high density lipoproteins (HDL) carry about 25 per cent of the blood cholesterol. In contrast to the usual cholesterol, which is low density lipoprotein (LDL) cholesterol and is harmful, the HDL cholesterol constitutes an antirisk factor and is beneficial to the heart. The higher the HDL cholesterol level, the better.

Regular exercise lowers elevated blood pressure, increases the beneficial HDL-cholesterol levels in the blood and thus protects the heart from attacks. A small daily intake of alcohol has also the same effect, while cigarette smoking depresses the HDL level. That may be one of the ways by which cigarettes exert their harmful effect on the heart. However, the mechanism involved in producing these effects is not yet clear.

Exercise has an important role in opening up collateral coronary channels which bypass the obstructions in the coronary arteries (chapter 4).

While physical exercise is good for the heart, we must understand clearly what exercise to do and how much. Too strenuous or unaccustomed exercise can be dangerous to the elderly people. Some even have dropped dead due to overexertion.

In such a situation, what and how much exercise do you advise for the elderly?

As a simple principle, we have to live our age. Football and hockey may provide an excellent form of exercise at 20 but not at 50. After the age of 40 any exercise that causes undue or unduly prolonged breathlessness, or a feeling of tiredness or pain in the chest even for a few minutes must not be indulged in. In fact, at any point of time you should not be forcing yourself to exercise. Any unaccustomed exercise must not be undertaken in the beginning. You must first accustom yourself to the exercise and its intricacies.

How should I go about doing this?

You should start with small bits of exercise and gradually increase the quantity. Attune yourself over days and weeks to perform more and more exercise. Once so attuned, continue, this trend. By and large, walking is the best form of exercise in the advancing years, starting at a slow pace and covering a small distance. Gradually increase your pace and speed as well as the distance walked. The easiest way to measure the distance of your walk is by the use of your watch.

If I have evidence of ischaemic heart disease, would you still advise me to exercise?

Yes, but all patients with known heart disease or those above the age of 55, and all persons above the age of 40 who have multiple risk factors for IHD, such as smoking, diabetes and hypertension, should consult their physicians before embarking on an exercise programme. The physician may submit you to exercise stress testing to find out your baseline stamina and the amount of exercise that will be safe for you as a starting point.

How much walking do you advise?

The important point is that at any point of time, when you are building up the quantum of your exercise, you should feel exhilarated after the exercise and not out of breath or unduly tired. At no time you should be forcing yourself to go on. If you gradually build up the tempo your capacity to exercise will increase without adverse effects. As a general rule, if you are able to achieve 30-45 minutes of brisk walking on five days a week, it should be adequate. Reserve the first five minutes for warming up and the last five minutes for cooling down.

What about active games such as tennis and badminton?

Such games should be played only for the sake of exercise and recreation, but never with the spirit of competition by the elderly.

The motto for the elderly: LIVE YOUR AGE.

Stress

It was about 25 years ago that I met an acquaintance of mine after a long gap. On a casual inquiry about his posting, I was surprised to learn that he had retired the previous month, meaning thereby that he had completed 58 years of age. As a doctor I am used to assessing the age of my patients and I had, in my mind, not placed him beyond the late forties. He looked at least 10 years younger than his age and was in excellent health. I was curious to know the reasons behind his lasting youth. He told me that during his service career of more than 30 years, he was always lucky to get good bosses as well as good subordinates to work with, and never had any problems with either. In fact, his mental make-up was such that he never got himself into conflicts. He kept himself relaxed, worked reasonably hard and remained in good health. He is now in his eighties, still alive and going strong.

I also know of an engineer, a brilliant inventor, who resigned his job to start his own consultancy work. An extremely ambitious man, he was always working against time and encountering obstacles. He suffered the first heart attack at 50, but refused to change his hectic life-style and died of another heart attack at 53. He literally drove himself to death.

These are two contrasting personalities; the former which is relaxed, keeps the heart attacks away and prolongs life; the latter tense, overly anxious and ambitious and working against time, driving a man towards heart problems and finally death.

What should be the mental attitude during the later years of life?

In the later years of your life you have to live your age, not only physically but also mentally and emotionally. You should have attained your ambitions by then. But if this is not the case, there is no use fretting over it or continue making half-hearted efforts. It is much better and saner to accept reality. Ambitions in old age need to be consistent with your physical, mental and psychological capacity.

Are you suggesting a life of inactivity in old age?

No, far from that, I am suggesting an active life till the end, but one which is within your capacity, with reasonable periods of rest and recreation. I am suggesting you keep a relaxed attitude of mind. What is important is not to work against time, not to be in a hurry, not to be too much timebound, not to look at your watch too often; in fact, to attempt to go in for a little more leisurely pace of work and activity with calm and composure without losing your temper. In other words, don't be at loggerheads with yourself. Be your own friend. To this end meditation may help.

How does meditation help?

Relaxation by the Indian technique of meditation is becoming increasingly popular, not only in our own country but also in the West. It is practised in many different forms: e.g., transcendental meditation of Maharishi Mahesh Yogi, made famous by the Beatles; and *Siddha* meditation, a slightly different variation practised by the followers of Swami Muktananda.

The principle of meditation is to use a mental device, which may be a mantra, a single word or a visual symbol, to relax the mind. From this bodily relaxation will flow. In effect, it means giving the mind something fairly unexciting to think about to blot out distracting thoughts. When such a thought enters the mind, it is replaced by the mantra, the single word or the visual symbol.

The technique is best learnt in a meditation centre. Many such centres are now functioning in almost all the big towns in India and abroad.

Food

Indian food mainly comprises carbohydrates, some fats and small amounts of proteins. Most Indians are fond of eating animal fat, derived mainly from milk in the form of *ghee* and butter. Only economic considerations prevent many Indians from consuming more. Fried foods such as *parathas, purees* and *samosa* are enjoyed all over north India and, therefore, consumed in plenty. A large percentage of the population is completely vegetarian due to religious beliefs. The so-called non-vegetarians are also vegetarian for the most part as a result of economic compulsions.

Which foods contribute towards the development of ischaemic heart disease?

Fats from animal source—*ghee*, butter, *malai* (cream), egg yolk (yellow part of the egg)— have a high content of saturated fat and cholesterol,and, therefore, contribute heavily towards the development of IHD. Egg yolk is particularly rich in cholesterol.

Refined sugar is being suspected as a serious risk factor for the heart, but clear evidence to this effect is still lacking.

What do you advise as a suitable cooking medium?

Vegetable oils, which are low in saturated fats but high in mono- or polyunsaturated fats. Any oil that does not solidify in the north Indian winter is suitable. However, the better ones are soyabean oil (Vital, Surya, Teacher brands), corn oil (Cornolla), sunflower and safflower oil (Saffola). Apart from the vegetable oils, certain fish oils are very useful in reducing blood cholesterol, but they are not available for general consumption in India. The vegetable oils are not only low in cholesterol but they also tend to reduce the cholesterol manufactured by the body.

Any particular problems in the use of vegetable oils as a cooking medium?

Chronic allergic reactions are not uncommon when vegetable oils are used. The reactions appear in the form of itching, stuffy nose, cough and sputum, and diarrhaea. These symptoms need not necessarily appear soon after a particular oil has begun being used, but may appear after weeks or months of use. When this happens the oil must be changed.

What is the role of salt?

A high salt intake contributes to the production of high blood pressure. Communities consuming a low salt diet habitually show lesser incidence of hypertension, which is an adverse factor for the heart.

What is the role of chillies and spices?

The role of chillies and spices has never been properly highlighted. The greater the quantity of these substances in the food, the great is the quantity of salt consumed. You cannot eat highly spiced food without putting a lot of salt in it. The more the quantity of chillies and the more the salt content, higher the blood pressure. In this context, it is necessary to mention that pickles (*achars*) and chutneys, which contain extra heavy amounts of salt, are relished by some people who consume large quantities.

If you are a hypertensive, you would be well advised to stop using chillies, spices, pickles and chutneys. You will find you can do with much less salt.

What is the role of fruits?

That high blood pressure is caused not only by high salt (sodium) intake but by low potassium intake is being increasingly recognised as an important factor. Potassium in our diet comes from fruits, particularly the citrus fruits (orange, *malta, mussammi*) and bananas. High intake of fruits with low salt intake, so as to keep a balance between sodium and potassium, is the correct course of action, especially for hypertensive patients.

Which is a better diet, vegetarian or non-vegetarian?

Not very long ago, vegetarians were considered second-rate human beings and generally inferior in health status. It is now being increasingly recognised that the vegetarian diet is healthier and that non-vegetarians, in general, have a lesser span of life than the vegetarians because of the former's increased susceptibility to heart attacks, and because vegetarian diet provides most of the antioxidants which are protective against free radicals.

What are free radicals and antioxidants?

Oxygen-free radicals, which are formed as a byproduct of cell metabolism and exposure of the body to sunlight and environmental pollutants like smoke of tobacco and automobiles, play havoc by destroying body cells. They are believed to be at the root of the aging process, heart attacks, strorkes, cancers, cataracts, etc.

Recent research has shown that a group of vitamins-A, C and E—offset the devastating effect of free radicals by neutralizing them. They are called antioxidants.

Betacarotene, the chemical parent of vitamin A, is found in dark green leafy vegetables, yellow and orange vegetables and fruits; Vitamin C in citrus fruits, green peppers, cabbage, and green leafy vegetables; vitamin E is found in whole grain, nuts, seeds and vegetable oils.

Even more improtant than vitamins for their role in the prevention of heart disease are phytochemicals—carotenoids and flavonoids—found in plant-based foods. Carotenoids are found in orange coloured vegetables, and flavonoids in many vegetable foods, including onions, broccoli, grape-skins, and tea (both green and black). Phytochemicals act as antioxidants and thus afford protection to the heart.

You can now appreciate how important the vegetarian diet is to health and well being.

On the whole, therefore, what diet do you recommend, especially to the elderly and to those who have already suffered a heart attack?

A mixed diet containing a wide variety of foodstuffs comprising the following:

- Vegetarian food, generally, including antioxidant cantaining items.
- Animal food, occasionally, as a good source of proteins.
- Fish (no bar to consumption).
- Fair amount of milk and yoghurt (curd), with most of the fat skimmed off, as a source of protein for the vegetarians.
- Vegetable oil (soyabean, corn, sunflower, safflower) as a cooking medium, in limited quantity.
- Sparse consumption of *ghee* and butter.
- Eggs, preferably avoid consumption, but, if not possible, not more than 5 per week.
- Pulses in plenty, as a source of proteins.

- Low salt, low spice and minimum chillies in the food; sparse use of pickles and chutneys (especially for hypertensives).
- plenty of fresh vegetables, fruits and salads.

If one has diabetes, what food do you advise for such a person?

The above mentioned diet with the following restrictions:

- No sugar.
- No sweets.
- Limited amounts of carbohydrates, equitably distributed during the day (the main sources of carbohydrates in our food are: rice, wheat bread and *chapatis,* root vegetables such as potato, sweet fruit such as mangoes and bananas and, of course, sugar and sweet dishes). The exact amount of carbohydrates to be consumed can be calculated by your doctor or dietician according to your height and weight and any reduction of body weight called for in case of obesity.
- Limited amounts of vegetable fats.

Beverages

Tea, coffee and alcohol in various forms are the common beverages consumed in our country. It is, therefore, important to examine their individual effects on the heart.

Is alcohol injurious to the heart?

Yes, alcohol is injurious to the heart as it is to the rest of the body, particularly to the stomach and the liver. However, in small quantities it may prove advantageous to the heart (1) by raising the levels of HDL cholesterol (which is an anti-risk factor for the heart) in blood (see section on Exercise), and (2) by providing a gentle tranquilising effect.

I have been a teetotaller all my life. If small quantities of alcohol are beneficial to the heart, should I start drinking?

No, even though alcohol is beneficial to the heart in small quantities, no doctor would advocate teetotallers to start drinking for the simple reason that this effect can be better achieved by other means, e.g., regular exercise. Secondly, even in small quantities, alcohol does adversely affect the body. Thirdly, it delays body reflexes while driving and contributes to road accidents. Lastly, the most serious problem regarding alcohol is that nobody can predict which person on starting alcohol consumption will become a compulsive drinker, i.e., an alcoholic.

To those who drink, what is the quantity of alcohol that you recommend?

A. Less than 50 ml of spirits like whisky or 500 ml of beer. Any quantity more than this will be neither beneficial to the heart nor safe for the liver and stomach. Keep two days in a week alcohol-free for reparative processes to take effect.

Are tea and coffee harmful?

A. In moderation tea and coffee are harmless. Tea, in addition, contains flavonoids which are antioxidants and protect the heart. These beverages give a lot of satisfaction to many people. They stimulate the body and remove the feeling of tiredness, but at the same time they also stimulate the heart rate. The effect of coffee is stronger due to its higher caffeine content. In consequence, the heart beats faster. Too much stimulation of the heart is not good for persons suffering from ischaemic heart disease and those in the older age group. Secondly, the sugar content of these beverages adds calories to the diet. You have to, therefore, strike a balance by observing moderation in tea or coffee consumption.

What exactly do you mean by 'moderation'?

In moderation tea and coffee are harmless. Tea, in addition, contains flavonoids which are antioxidants and protect the heart.

By moderation I mean avoid consumption of very strong tea and coffee; do not consume too much at a time; and do not drink these beverages late in the evenings if they tend to disturb your sleep. Good sleep is important for proper recuperation after a day's work. This is particularly true for the elderly. On an average three or four cups of less than average strength tea and an occasional cup of coffee, with minimum amount of sugar, should prove both satisfying and harmless.

Work and Recreation

Some reduction in physical capacity after a heart attack and a gradual decline due to advancing years are inevitable. What adjustments one should make regarding work and recreation after a heart attack shall be discussed in the chapters to follow. Here we shall discuss what ought to be done as age advances.

What precautions are necessary regarding the performance of work as the years go by?

Up to the age of about 50, the physical capacity remains almost unimpaired, unless some mishap like a heart attack occurs. Beyond 50, the capacity to do physical work gradually, but surely, starts declining. The speed as well as the quantum of physical work should therefore be gradually toned down, so that after a day's work you do not feel fagged out or excessively tired.

Are any precautions necessary while doing mental work?

The capacity to do mental work normally remains unimpaired till late in life, though the capacity for the physical component of the work, i.e., reaching the place of work, obtaining the mode of transport, sitting on a chair for certain specified hours, becomes less and less as age advances. Hence, such factors as the distance travelled, the type of transport (e.g., cycle vs. public bus vs. private car), the comfort offered by the chair in which you have to sit become more and more important as years pass by. If part of your work involves undue physical effort, you must arrange for assistance.

At first sight, these factors may appear to be too trivial to bother about, but constant tiresome, long journeys and uncomfortable place of sitting and working will inevitably take their toll. If you wish to continue working till late in life, which you should for a comfortable living and healthy mental attitude, make yourself as comfortable as possible on the above scores.

If hard work can produce problems in old age, would it not be correct to give up active work altogether?

No, one should try and remain active as long as possible in order to maintain physical and mental health and one's dignity. Inactivity is not conducive to good health, neither physical nor mental. Activity within one's capacity should be undertaken. However, long hours of continuous work should be avoided; there should be adequate periods of rest in between.

What about recreation?

Recreation is equally essential, but it also demands more physical effort or less depending upon its nature. Recreation should be such that it is not too much of a drain on the limited energy available. It has become fashionable these days to advocate almost unlimited physical activity for old people including those who have sustained a myocardial infarction. The pendulum has swung far too much from almost complete inertia to unlimited physical activity. It is time we realise that the physical activity is beneficial to a certain extent, but when the limits are exceeded it can prove really harmful. Therefore, too strenuous recreational activity, skiing for example, may be left to the younger people to enjoy. Cinema, theatre, television, reading and writing for pleasure, non-competitive games are the activities to indulge in. Holidaying should be comfortable and enjoyable. If in the hills, climbing steep heights should be avoided.

Drugs

Are there any drugs to prevent heart attacks?

Yes, the use of aspirin in small daily doses has already been mentioned in Chapter 7. Recent work suggests that antioxidant vitamins A, C and E are also useful in this respect in daily doses of 5000 units, 150 mg and 65 mg respectively.

12

Life after a Heart Attack

Congratulations on your wonderful recovery from a heart attack. You are now up and about after the convalescent period. It takes about six months for nature's repair processes to take full effect. Your doctor would have assessed the amount of damage suffered by your heart muscle, its repair and progress, the present status of the heart and its exercise tolerance. There is now no reason for despondency. People have lived for 25 years or more after a heart attack and have lived well. Only a bit of care and some precautions are necessary to ensure longevity and a trouble-free life in the future.

Can my neart function as long as it would have done had there been no heart attack?

Certainly; it is not only possible, but you can make it happen. Let me tell you a true story first.

Thirty years ago I purchased a shaving mirror, a small beautiful round piece, and I loved it. Unfortunately my small son cracked a corner soon after purchase. I felt unhappy, repaired it with araldite and started reusing it. Since I loved the piece, I became doubly cautious in handling it. I still have that mirror and it is as useful today as it was 30 years ago. I am sure, if it had not been damaged, I would not have given it the extra care that I did and it would have long ago disappeared.

Similarly, your heart has survived an injury. Nature has healed it. With due care and by observing some precautions you can make it last for a long period probably longer than if nothing had happened to it. These precautions mentioned here and in the following chapters, are simple and easy to follow.

What is the most important precaution?

The most important question is how much work load should one put on one's heart? The answer is simple: the amount of work which does not cause any problem by way of adverse symptoms of chest pain, shortness of breath, undue tiredness or weakness or palpitations. This is the golden rule, which is to be always observed. Within the framework of this rule whatever fits in is right, whatever does not is wrong.

Doctor, are you suggesting a life of inactivity?

No, far from it. This golden rule does not mean inactivity at all. On the contrary, physical activity is good for the heart. As already stated, it increases the HDL- cholesterol levels of the blood which is an anti-risk factor for the heart. The higher the HDL level, the better. Regular exercise is therefore, good for you.

All that you have to learn is how best to perform the maximum possible activity and yet not cross your limit.

What if I am obese?

If you are obese, even a small amount of work or exercise may produce adverse symptoms. Hence, the important thing you have to do is to shed some of your weigh and come down to your ideal weight level or below it. Instructions in this regard have already been given in the previous chapter in the section on 'Obesity'.

My tolerance to exercise is low. What is the best way to increase it?

Your exercise tolerance at the moment may be low. You are probably a sedentary worker and have not been in the habit of performing regular exercise. To be able to lead a life involving normal activity and work, you have to increase your exercise tolerance. The only way to achieve this objective is to gradually increase the amount and intensity of exercise. The best form of exercise for you to start with is walking on the level. Using your watch walk at a moderate pace and note the number of minutes you are able to walk comfortably without developing any of the adverse symptoms mentioned above. This is your starting point. Go on adding to it 1-2 minutes on alternate days till you reach your maximum limit or one hour of walking. At any point while increasing your walking time, if you encounter adverse symptoms, decrease the time of walking by a couple of minutes for a few days and then start increasing it again. When you are able to walk freely on the level, start increasing your speed and the distance walked. Once you have reached your maximum speed and distance on the level, try climbing stairs, a few steps at first, adding one or two steps at a time on alternate days, and go on increasing the number of steps to reach the maximum, i.e., when you can climb without any adverse symptoms. The same principles apply to cycling, going uphill, or for that matter, any exercise or work. Once you have reached your maximum level of physical activity, keep it up.

The important point is never to force yourself to go on exercising in the face of adverse symptoms or when you are too tired. Another important point is never to undertake unaccustomed exercise or work. Accustom yourself first and know your limits of tolerance and adhere to them. In this context, you will appreciate the fact that any sudden, severe spurt of activity, physical or emotional, can be dangerous for your heart and must, therefore, be avoided at all costs. For the same reason, any game or sport in which you are likely to overshoot your limits should not be indulged in. Competitive games are, therefore, out of the question. However, they may be played strictly with the aim of deriving fun and exercise.

After you have attained your maximum level of exercise tolerance, it is quite possible that you may be amazed to find yourself capable of performing previously unimaginable amounts of exercise and activity.

Doctor, do I have to take some medicines as a measure of prevention?

Your doctor would have prescribed some medication to protect your heart from undue strain (e.g., betablocking drugs) and also to inhibit the formation of blood clots in the coronary arteries (e.g., aspirin). These drugs have been found useful in reducing your chances of developing reinfarction.

How long do these medicines have to be taken?

These drugs have to be continued indefinitely under the care of your physician.

Are there any precautions to be taken because this is a long-term therapy?

Yes, the betablockers should never be abruptly stopped. You must replenish stocks in time, so that there is no default whatsoever.

The aspirin should be taken in a soluble form (disprin) and the dosage not more than 1/2 tablet daily dissolved in a glass of water soon after meals. This will prevent its irritating effect on the stomach which can cause ulcer and bleeding from the stomach. It should be remembered that increasing the dose of aspirin leads to a loss of its beneficial effect on the heart and increases the chances of bleeding from the stomach. In effect, 50-150 mg of aspirin per day is enough. Enteric coated tablets (e.g. ASA-50, Laprin-75 and 150; Ecosprin-75 & 150) which do not injure the stomach and do not need to be dissolved are available.

When do I need to report to my doctor?

Apart from regular check ups, beware of the warning symptoms like:

- pain in the chest, arm
- breathlessness,

- earache or toothache without a local cause,
- a feeling of lump in the throat on exertion, and
- palpitations and irregular pulse and heart beat.

If at any time any of these symptoms appear, report to your doctor immediately, especially if adequate doses of nitroglycerine cannot control them. Do not, under any circumstances, try out any other drug.

What are the other measures you suggest in my case by way of prevention?

All the measures suggested in the chapter on 'Prevention' (Chapter 10) are doubly applicable to you. To summarize:

- No smoking.
- No chewing of tobacco in any form including *pan* and *pan masala.*
- If you drink, take alcohol in strict moderation of one peg a day and never exceed two.
- Reduce your weight to lower than the ideal level.
- Avoid sweets and too much carbohydrates and fats, so that you do not gain weight.
- Do not consume any animal fats (*ghee,* butter, *malai,* yolk of egg, organ meat) if your blood cholesterol is above 220 mg per cent.
- Use vegetable oils as cooking medium—oils which do not solidify in the north Indian winter.
- Take a vegetarian diet as far as possible with plenty of fresh green vegetables and fresh fruits.
- Avoid red meat (lamb or beef); fish is excellent; white meat is acceptable.
- If you have high blood pressure, take a low salt diet (one-third or less of the usual consumption); proper control of BP under the directions of your physician is imperative.
- If you have diabetes, further restriction on your diet, as suggested in chapter 10 and Appendix should be enforced. Proper control of the condition under the guidance of your physician is of paramount importance.

- Remember that the control of both hypertension and diabetes, is a lifelong process.
- Maintain regular hours of work, meals, rest and recreation, so that there are no periods of sudden or excessive strain.
- Stop working against time; avoid hurry; stop looking at your watch too often; feel free and easy-going rather than being too much time-bound.
- Keep your cool; avoid losing your temper.
- In other words maintain steady and moderate pace of life physically, mentally and emotionally without hurry or tension.

Sexual activity after a heart attack has not been discussed in this chapter. This important subject is dealt with separately in Chapter13.

13

Limitations after a Heart Attack

After recovering from a heart attack, the patient would like to know the limitations, if any, imposed on his freedom of movement, the prospects of his rejoining duty at the place of his work, the restrictions on the games that he would like to play, exercise that he would like to do and holidays that he would like to enjoy. Can he go to the hills in summer on a vacation? Can he fly to Europe on his business tour? Can he indulge in sex as he used to? These are the questions whose answers an average patient would like to know as early as possible after recovery from a heart attack.

The answers to all the questions posed above depend upon two fundamental points—how much damage has been inflicted on the heart muscle and what is or will be the ultimate physical status of the heart? In simple terms this means how much physical exertion the heart can withstand. There is no doubt that the greater the damage, the lesser is the physical reserve of the heart and the lesser the ability to withstand the stresses and strains of life. Within this framework the physician has to advise the patient on the questions posed above.

There is no doubt that your physician will do his best to restore your maximum level of physical fitness, and, if you cooperate with him, and gradually increase your exercise tolerance as suggested in the previous chapter, you may be amazed to find the level of physical fitness that you can attain.

I will now answer the questions posed above, except that sexual activity after a heart attack has been dealt with separately in the next chapter.

Will I be able to go back to my old job?

This is a very crucial question, on which depend the bread and butter of the family. It has been repeatedly found that the best job for a heart attack patient is that job which he had been doing all his life, where productivity is likely to be maximum with minimum of effort. This is true whether you are a self-employed person or an employee. In this context, it could be stated with confidence that at least four out of five persons who have had a heart attack can ultimately return to their old jobs. An all-out effort should be made with the cooperation of the employer as well as fellow employees to make the patient adjust to his old job or, at least at his old place of work, with the nature of duties duly changed, if necessary, to suit the changed physical condition of the patient. The least difficulty in this respect is likely to be experienced in the case of desk workers or others whose job does not involve much physical work. It is in the case of manual workers that adjustment could create some difficulty. It is usually not difficult in the public sector or government service, where, generally, the people are more accommodating for the simple reason that they are all employees. In the private sector real difficulties may sometimes be experienced, because the private employer has to pay from his own pocket, and he, therefore, demands the worth of his money. In any case, it is always worthwhile exploring the possibilities of a more suitable job for the patient without harming the interest of the employer. In a small number of cases it may become necessary to advise a change of job, because the present job would be so demanding physically that the patient's state of health would not permit.

When can I drive my car/scooter?

Most people nowadays depend on their personal means of transport for commuting to and from their place of work. A personal car or scooter does save a lot of time and inconvenience, but driving on the busy and congested roads of towns and metropolitan cities involves a high degree of tension. Consequently, the heart rate at times goes up considerably. This can strain the heart. Much also depends upon the attitude of the person driving the vehicle. If he enjoys driving and keeps himself relaxed, then the tension and the consequent rise in heart rate are much less. But if he loses his temper and is at his nerves' end, then the pulse rate would jump up to much higher level. All these factors will have to be taken into consideration before allowing a patient to drive his own vehicle. In general terms, most patients would find it safe to drive a vehicle six to twelve months after a heart attack, if there are no other complications.

When can I undertake an aeroplane flight?

This question should be divided into two parts—domestic flights and international flights. The former are relatively short distance flights without the distressing immigration and customs formalities, though the security checks have become equally cumbersome now. A patient would, therefore, be fit to undertake a domestic journey by air much earlier than international travel. The loss of atmospheric pressure at the high altitudes at which the aircrafts fly poses no problem because the modern aircrafts are fully pressurised. The considerations are the length of the journey, the conditions at the airports of entry and exit, the necessity of carrying heavy luggage, inconvenient timings from country to country and problems of food and rest. While a domestic flight may be undertaken after a month or two of recovery from an uncomplicated heart attack, it may have to be much longer, about a year, before the patient can be considered fit for international flights. It must be admitted that the tolerance to undergo privation and inconvenience as a result of long travel is lowered after a heart attack. This fact has to be kept in mind when the patient wants to go abroad. If after a test flight the patient does not feel too well, he should avoid such flights in future.

When can I take part in games?

While exercise is good for the heart, excessive exercise can be dangerous. Games, therefore, should be played strictly with the idea of deriving fun and exercise. All competitive games are prohibited after a heart attack. Your physician can advise you, after checking your exercise tolerance, when precisely you should start playing games, lighter ones first, and more strenuous ones later.

What sort of exercise is ideal for me?

This aspect has been discussed in detail in the previous chapter.

Is sex life over for me? If not, when can I indulge in sex? Any precautions to be taken?

No, sex life is not over for you. This is a very important question and has, therefore, been discussed in a separate chapter which follows.

I want to go on a pilgrimage to Vaishnodevi, which is located in the hills near Jammu. When can I go?

You must reach that state of physical fitness in which you can tolerate the rail and bus travel as well as travel by pony and on foot, and also be able to wait in a queue for an almost indefinite amount of time. It will take some months, or may be a year, before such a state can be attained provided the damage to your heart muscle has not been extensive and there have been no complications. Your physician will evaluate your fitness for such a venture by examining your exercise tolerance.

Similarly, going on Haj will entail travel by air or ship to Mecca, local travel by taxi and on foot. The same remarks as above apply to the pilgrimage for Haj.

What about holidays in the hills?

Apart from the travel, special considerations with respect to the hills are the height above the sea level, the necessity to go uphill and downhill on foot, and prohibition on plying cars and buses within the municipal limits of the hill station. As the height from sea level increases, the atmospheric pressure falls and can lead to a lack of oxygen in the body, which is not good for the heart patient. Up to about 5000 feet above sea level this effect is not pronounced, but above that height, it would be inadvisable for the patient to go for a holiday. It would be preferable to choose a location where there are level walks nearby rather than a place marked by steep ascents or descents. Further, it would be wise to let a day or two be reserved for acclimatisation before undertaking strenuous trips on foot. Of course, your undertaking a trip to the hills will arise only after you have recovered fully and achieved a satisfactory degree of exercise tolerance. For this purpose about a year should be allowed after a heart attack.

What about my social life?

Your social life may have to be readjusted. As stated above, your tolerance to undergo privations and inconveniences would have decreased after a heart attack. You will be better off with fixed routines which have been carefully planned and tailored to meet your health status with proper timings for rest and recreation. As far as possible fit in your social engagements into this routine. Making long and inconvenient trips to fulfill social obligations on marriages, births and deaths should be avoided as far as possible.

14

Sexual Activity after a Heart Attack

Discussion on matters of sex has been considered and still continues to be taboo in India even though it profoundly affects the personal life of each one of us. Even today, most patients are reluctant to ask questions on this crucial topic and most doctors are equally reluctant to offer advice. This results in much avoidable fear and suffering not only for the patients but also for their spouses.

Let me narrate an incident which occurred about ten years ago when such suffering was prevented by timely advice.

A fifty-year-old patient of mine, who had recently recovered from a heart attack, came to consult me. He said that a distant uncle, who had come to see him, had told him that his sex life was now over and that it would be dangerous for him to indulge in sex any more. He had been a rather active 'player' in the game of sex all his life. He was naturally very upset and worried and had come to consult me on this very issue. It was more than three months since he had sustained myocardial infarction, and by this time he had recovered fully. His exercise tolerance was good and there was no disturbance of the heart rhythm nor any other complication. Accordingly I advised him to resume sex with his wife forthwith. More than ten years have passed. He has been happy and there have been no heart problems attributable to sex. This is a typical case and there are innumerable such cases who were encouraged to enjoy sex life after a heart attack, after they had been brought to a level of physical fitness where it would not only be safe but desirable to resume normal sex life.

Unfortunately, the fear psychosis among some of the patients and their spouses is so deep that sometimes a lot of persuasions is required to make patients resume this activity. It is very common for patients not to receive any advice from their doctors, or to receive a very guarded one which, in effect, is of little value.

Can every patient resume sexual activity after a heart attack?

Almost 80-90 per cent of patients should be able to do so sooner or later.

Who are the patients who can resume the activity earlier?

All those patients who have recovered without complications and have no abnormality of the rhythm of the heart and whose exercise tolerance is good.

What exercise tolerance do you rate as good?

A patient who can go up and down the Master's stool 15-20 times each way at a good speed, or can generate 75 watt on a bicycle ergometer, without producing angina, arrhythmia or undue breathlessness or adverse changes in his electrocardiogram, is fit to resume normal sex life. As a rough indication, the ability to go up a flight of stairs at a good speed without producing any of the adverse symptoms enumerated above is good enough for normal sex.

How long does it take to reach such a state of fitness after the attack?

Anywhere from eight to twelve weeks after an uncomplicated heart attack. Of course, it would take longer if the infarction were more extensive and accompanied by complications.

What do you advise if exertion produces adverse symptoms?

Such cases will have to be individually assessed. The requisite advice will depend upon their health status and the degree of control of symptoms through medication. For example, if a patient gets anginal pain after sex and if the angina can be prevented by suitable medication (usually nitrates) taken before the act and no other adverse symptoms or disturbances of heart rhythm are noticed, such a patient may be allowed the pleasure of sexual intercourse. But if, on the other hand, dangerous disturbances of heart rhythm are produced by exertion or if the patient has chronic left ventricular failure, it will be prudent for him to avoid the exertion of sex till better times.

Can the sex act precipitate a fresh heart attack?

Studies have shown that in the course of normal daily activities, there are plenty of circumstances during which the heart rate rises considerably to as high as or higher than during normal sexual activity, for instance, during driving a scooter in a crowded, traffic-infested market place. The risk of precipitating a heart attack during normal sexual intercourse is, therefore, no greater than during other daily activities. But what is important are the circumstances attendant on the sexual intercourse.

What are these circumstances and why are they important?

Sexual activity carried out in the confines of the home in the marital bed with a sympathetic wife as the partner is just another normal human function. Contrast this with clandestine sex in a hotel room with a strange partner with whom one's potency has to be proved. Also there could have been lot of smoking and drinking prior to the act. Further, the anxiety and fear of being found out coupled with feeling of guilt could make matters worse. All these factors produce a much greater strain. Naturally, the chances of precipitating a heart attack under these circumstances become much higher.

Can sudden death take place during intercourse?

Yes it is possible, but most such deaths have occurred under clandestine circumstances for the reasons cited above. The probability of a fresh heart attack or sudden death during sexual intercourse at home under normal circumstances is no greater than in any other normal day-to-day activity.

Any precautions that you advise?

Avoid intercourse soon after meals. Wait for at least four hours after a meal, which is the time required for digestive processes to take place when a lot of blood is diverted for this purpose, leaving less for the use of the heart.

Secondly, if certain positions are too strenuous and precipitate symptoms like breathlessness or chest pain, change the position to a less strenuous one and let your partner play the more active role.

Use of viagra in heart patients can he dangerous, particularly in those who are taking nitrates (Angised, Sorbitrate). It can cause a sudden and dangerous fall of blood pressure in them.

Do you advise the use of any drugs to protect the heart during intercourse?

Cardioprotective drugs such as betablockers are usually advised after a heart attack. A tablet an hour or so before the act may prevent the heart rate from shooting up too high and thus prevent the possibility of a fresh attack or sudden death. This measure is especially important if hypertension coexists. Your doctor will be able to advise you the correct dose for you after making certain that there are no contraindications to their use.

Finally, what are your conclusions?

Normal healthy sexual activity at home with a loving and sympathetic spouse is to be encourged after a heart attack, provided there are no adverse factors and exercise tolerance is good. To start with, this activity may be kept at moderate, less-than-intense levels with the spouse acting as the active partner. As time passes the intensity can be gradually increased. Cardioprotective drugs (betablockers) may be used under the guidance of your physician.

15

Sex in the Elderly

A popular myth which has been going around in our country is that after the age of 50 for men and after menopause in women, all sex life comes to an end. While there is no doubt that as age advances, the physical capacity declines and so does the frequency of the sex act, it is certainly not true that after 50 there is no sex life.

Is there anything wrong in indulging in sexual activity by the elderly?

Unfortunately, in our country, the sex act has been equated with base and vulgar activities, and not looked upon as a normal human function like eating and working. Celibacy has been eulogised and put on a premium. The result is that the elderly couples feel guilty while indulging in normal sex life. The guilt complex may be responsible for a lot of marital unhappiness, because it may lead to unsatisfying sex. It is time that, we as a nation, realise that sexual activity within the confines of the home is like any other human activity. You can and should indulge in it without feeling guilty about it, at any age and to whatever extent your physical capacity and general health permit you.

Do you mean to say that there can be unrestrained sexual activity during the later years?

A normal sex life can and should be enjoyed during the later years of your life, though perhaps with a progressively decreasing frequency and intensity, provided both the husband and wife maintain good health, are capable of physical activity and possess the capacity. It should be remembered that a normal sex act demands a healthy body and a healthy mind.

How do you ensure this physical capacity?

Your physical capacity to a large extent depends upon the health of your heart and lungs. If you wish to continue enjoying sexual life till late in life, keep your heart in order and stay healthy. The chapter on 'Prevention' will help you to keep your heart and body healthy.

Are there any precautions to be observed?

The precautions necessary are broadly the same as for any other physical activity during the advancing years. Any activity which causes abnormal symptoms such as pain in the chest, breathlessness or undue weakness has to be avoided.

How frequent and how intense should the sex act be in the later years?

If, after the act, you attain a feeling of deep satisfaction and none of the adverse symptoms mentioned above occurs, the intensity and frequency are just right for you. But if such symptoms do occur you probably need to reduce the intensity and frequency of the act, as well as consult your physician for the cause and treatment of your symptoms. He will also advise you what exactly to do in the matter relating to your sex life.

There is no particular intensity or frequency of the sex act which can be laid down as a rule of thumb for the elderly. Individual capacities must be respected. Probably once, sometimes twice, a week at moderate intensity may suit most elderly couples in apparent good health.

Do you think infrequent sex act with long periods of abstinence is more suitable for the elderly?

No, long periods of abstinence followed by sexual activity are not advisable for two reasons. First, such periods of abstinence are invariably followed by too intense sexual activity. Secondly, the partners may become unaccustomed to the activity. Such unaccustomed intense activity can be harmful. This situation would be similar to an old man running a race at full speed after remaining inactive for a month. No, it would be much saner for the elderly to remain accustomed to moderate, less-than-intense sex activity rather than maintain long periods of abstinence punctuated by occasional bursts of intense sexual activity.

Do you advise any medication for overcoming sluggish sexual activity?

Stimulation of sexual activity in later years can be dangerous, because you will tend to overshoot your capacity. Also, there are really no effective and, at the same time, safe drugs available for the purpose. Use of viagra (when available in India) can be dangerous in old age by stimulating the sexual appetite to undesirable levels. Viagra combined with clandestine sex in an elderly person can prove to be a lethal combination. Avoid it. A normal person needs no drugs to stimulate his sex drive. If you find your sex drive waning, consult your doctor for the cause and its treatment.

What about hormones?

The same remarks as above apply to hormones.

16

IHD Families

There are families in which ischaemic heart disease is common and heart attacks occur at an early age. It is important to know why this happens and what can be done to help prevent the disease in unaffected younger members of these families.

What is the usual age after which a heart attack is not unexpected?

As age advances, fatty deposits occur in the coronary arteries and by the age of about 60 almost everyone is presumed to have some atheromatous lesions in his/her coronary arteries. Hence myocardial infarction occurring after the age of about 55 is not an unexpected event, but one occurring before that is.

What happens in families prone to have heart attacks?

The attacks occur at an early age when the members of these families are still in their thirties or forties. Younger the age, severer the attack.

Why do attacks occur at an early age?

Many factors can be responsible. Their lipid profile may be faulty; total and LDH-cholesterol may be high and/or the beneficial HDL-cholesterol too low. Triglycerides too may be high. Their blood may be more easily coagulable. Obesity in these families is common. While the lipid abnormalities may be genetic in origin, their diet is usually faulty and rich in animal fat, and overeating is common. In some families, diabetes is common and may be the factor responsible for early IHD.

Why are the heart attacks in these families very severe?

I have explained in chapter 4 that collateral circulation which bypasses the atheromatous obstructions takes time to develop under natural conditions. If a heart attack occurs at an early age, there has not been enough time available for them to develop. The result is that in the event of complete obstruction occurring, say due to thrombosis in the artery, there is no alternative source of blood supply to the affected part of the heart and the attack becomes massive.

There can be another reason. The number of the fine intercommunicating channels, which become anastomotic channels, is genetically determined. In some families their number may be too small, so that effective collateral circulation does not develop.

What should be done by members of these families?

It is important for you to know your family history. In case some of the older members of your family have had heart attack or met with sudden unexpected death before the age of 55, it becomes important for the younger members to start taking precautions early in life. They should get their blood pressure, blood sugar and lipid profile checked regularly, say twice a year, and keep their blood pressure and/or diabetes under good control with the help of their physicians if any of these conditions is present in them. Secondly, they must not add any more risk factors to their lifestyle because their heredity is against them. In effect, lifestyle of the whole family should be changed to one of simple life in which smoking has no place, drinking is in strict moderation, there is no overeating, animal fats are avoided and a diet which is well balanced and generally vegetarian. The life should be physically active and obesity should be avoided. These precautions are the same as for anyone else but they should be strictly enforced, not on an individual but on the whole family, so that children learn and get used to such a life from a tender age. With these precautions, the members of these families can substantially reduce their risk of getting heart attacks.

17

Care of the Heart after Cardiac Surgery

After successful surgery of the heart, whether by-pass operation or the quasi-surgical procedure of angioplasty, the patient feels much better. His angina may be relieved and may even disappear. His need for antianginal drugs may markedly diminish. His exercise tolerance may increase considerably. He may feel that he is back to normal or near normal. Under these circumstances he may be tempted to continue the life-style he was accustomed to—smoking, drinking, eating.

Can he smoke with impunity? Can he drink alcohol in unlimited amounts? Can he eat as he likes? Can he indulge in sexual intercourse? How much exertion is allowed to him? These are some of the questions to which clear-cut answers are necessary.

To understand this, it is important to know what the operation does and what it does not do to the disease.

What does the by-pass operation do to the disease process?

It is important to realise that the by-pass operation does not and cannot remove the cause of the disease—the obstructing atheroma in the coronary artery. It merely bypasses the obstruction. The obstructing lesions remain where they were. In fact, with most of the blood now diverted through the bypass graft, the blood flow through the natural coronary arteries is further slowed down. This slowing down of the blood flow only tends to make the obstruction more complete. Secondly, the bypass graft, which is usually made out of a vein, is a much weaker structure than coronary artery and consequently more liable to develop obstruction by way of blood clot. The benefit of the operation therefore tends to wane six years or so (longer with arterial graft) after the operation. This is related to the closure of the bypass graft.

What does angioplasty do to the disease?

The operation presses down the atheroma and thus dilates the lumen of the coronay artery at the point of stenosis. It does not remove the atheroma. While the initial success rate may be as high as 75 to 90 per cent, the predominant problem is of restenosis. Almost one-third of the operated arteries restenose within six months, with return of symptoms needing redilatation or by-pass operation, though position has improved since insertion of stents was started.

Then, what do you advise me?

You would have appreciated by now that coronary bypass operation or angioplasty are not a panacea for IHD. They are merely some of the useful steps in the total care of the coronary patient. The lesson of the story is that after the operation you will have to continue to take all the preventive measures outlined in chapter 10 with as much vigour as you would if the operation had not been performed.

This answers all your questions on smoking, alcohol, diet, etc.

What about medical treatment?

Medical treatment of residual angina, if any, will be continued, though reduced to the extent necessary. The treatment of hypertension or diabetes, if co-existing, will also be continued on the lines already indicated. Aspirin as a preventive for heart attacks will also be continued. Recently, antioxidant vitamins A, C, and E (A & E in particular) have been shown to substantially reduce the incidence of heart attack along with beneficial effects on many other degenerative diseases.

How much physical activity can I indulge in?

Your exercise tolerance would have increased after you have recuperated from the operation. You should increase your level of physical activity accordingly, slowly building it up to the highest level possible without initiating symptoms of chest pain, breathlessness or undue tiredness. Build up your exercise tolerance as explained in chapter 11, and keep it up. It will keep the arteries patent longer.

What about sexual intercourse?

No problem; if your exercise tolerance is good and the act does not produce any adverse symptoms but a feeling of well being, you may resume sexual activity. Chapter 13 should guide you adequately in this regard.

18

Non-Cardiac Surgery in Heart Patients

Surgical operations for such conditions as enlarged prostate, gall bladder or kidney stones, removal of the uterus, etc., may be required to be done in a patient who has had a heart attack, or has angina. Are there any risks involved? What is to be done? How to ensure the safety of the patient? These are some of the questions which I will answer in this chapter.

Is it risky for patients of ischaemic heart disease to undergo surgical operations?

All major surgery does carry some element of risk, which is increased if IHD is present. But the risk is more under certain situations.

What are those situations?

Soon after myocardial infarction; disturbances of heart rhythm, failing function of the heart, and uncontrolled, severe or unstable angina pose special risks to the patient if he goes for major surgical operations.

What should be done after heart attack?

Wait for at least six months for major surgery after the attack, and longer, may be a year, if the attack was accompanied by complications. Exceptions are emergent operations e.g., serious road side accidents.

What if there are disturbances of heart rhythm?

They should be treated and controlled by your physician before you go for the operation. The control may be necessary during the operation.

What to do if there is failure of function of the heart?

This should also be well controlled by your physician. There should be no breathing difficulty and exercise tolerance at least fair before major surgery can be undertaken.

What about angina?

Angina should be well controlled. If angina is severe or unstable, operation should be postponed. But if for some reason it cannot be postponed, a revascularisation operation such as balloon angioplasty or bypass surgery may first be necessary before the non-cardiac operation is performed. Such a situation may occur rarely.

19

Cardiac Care of Aged Parents

Your parents may be in their seventies or eighties. Hypertension, angina, heart attacks, disturbances of heart rhythm and congestive heart failure are not uncommon at this age. Although general principles of heart care are the same as described in the book, some differences do exist. These variations should be known to you before you can give them proper care.

Why variations in care are necessary?

Priorities at this age are somewhat different. The first priority is to ensure, as far as possible, a good quality of life, rather than a mere addition of a few months or years to their life span.

In old age, diseases of other systems like the brain, kidneys, prostate, etc., and cancer are also common, and may interfere with a successful outcome of treatment which may have to be amended accordingly. For the same reason, certain cardiac operations and interventions may not be possible or desirable.

Disease or death of the spouse or a dear and near one may have serious repercussions on the old person's health by causing psychological imbalance, and may aggravate or precipitate malfunctioning of the heart. It is very necessary for you and your children to provide the surviving parent support and succour.

What are the variations?

In common with other body responses, which are slow, the elderly tend to suppress or minimise their symptoms. Even serious complaints may be mentioned only in the passing or not at all. A pain of heart attack may not be complained of or it may be actually painless and manifest only as profuse sweating and weakness. You and your doctor will have to be careful to give due weight to their complaints, which may sometimes be spoken only casually.

Sudden changes of temperature are ill tolerated by the elderly. Extreme cold or heat have a strong deleterious effect on their heart and may precipitate or aggravate angina, heart attack or congestive heart failure. They need to be protected against such exposure.

Many elderly patients are much disturbed when they are shifted from home to a hospital. This aggravates their illness, sometimes markedly. They should be treated, as far as possible, at home. They should be shifted to a hospital only if there is emergency and treatment is such that cannot be carried out at home.

Clearance of the drugs by the liver and kidneys of the old people is slow, with the result that your doctor will give smaller doses, less frequently and for a shorter period. This is particularly true of sedatives and tranquilizers. For the same reason, all unnecessary drugs are avoided. If you find any untoward effect, e.g., inattention or dizziness, report to your doctor immediately. Close monitoring by your doctor is necessary to prevent occurrence of side-effects of drugs. Some may have to be stopped as soon as improvement warrants or side-effects become troublesome.

While activity has to be encouraged, they should not indulge in strenuous exercise.

What are the aims of treatment which I should keep in view?

It is not always possible to cure an elderly person of his cardiac ailment, but it is certainly possible to give him good medical care so that he/she is able to spend his/her remaining years with best possible quality of life by making optimum use of his limited cardiac capacity. Making large-scale modifications in their diet and living pattern or submitting them to surgical or semisurgical interventions without regard to their ultimate outcome, are neither appreciated by the elderly nor they are desirable. There is no point in giving injudicious therapy or operations in an attempt to give a few months or years at the cost of quality of life. The primary aim should therefore be to ensure optimum quality of life rather than number of years, which should be secondary.

With these modifications, all the preventive measures mentioned in the book are as applicable to the elderly as to others.

20

Pseudo-cardiac Disorders

Fear of heart disease can induce untoward symptoms. A death in the family due to heart attack is not an uncommon cause for this fear. The introvert, maladjusted and neurotic individuals are particularly prone to such apprehensions.

What are the common symptoms?

The common symptoms are palpitations and chest pain of non-cardiac origin.

What are palpitations and how are they produced in normal people?

Palpitations are pounding or fluttering sensations in the heart region and are due to consciousness of heart action. Normally, people are unaware of their heart beat. However, normal people can experience palpitations at certain times; for example, after intense physical exercise or sexual intercourse, when the heart rate goes up considerably. But the maladjusted or neurotic individuals may experience the symptom at near normal rates of less than 100 per minute.

What are the abnormal ways in which palpitations are produced?

Palpitations can be experienced when the rhythm of the heart is disturbed or when its rate becomes too rapid. These disturbances of rhythm may be the result of some organic disease of the heart, or they may occur without a known cause. This is especially true of extrasystoles (extra beats) which can appear with or without an underlying heart disease, and can be precipitated by such items of food as tea or coffee. While some patients may not even be aware of their existence, others may experience distressing fluttering sensations with no underlying heart disease to account for it. Consequently, the fear of heart disease may become intense.

What are the main characteristics of non-cardiac chest pain?

The main distressing symptom is the chest pain or pain in the shoulder or arm. Any pain occurring in this region, especially on the left side of the chest, can cause much anxiety about the safety of the heart in susceptible individuals. On the other hand, a serious cardiac pain of low intensity may be ignored by the patient, causing serious delay in starting the treatment and thus putting his life in jeopardy.

The chest pains of non-cardiac origin particularly generate anxiety when they occur on the left side of the chest because heart is located on this side. The pain may be fixed at one spot which may be tender on applying pressure. Movements of the chest wall or of the upper limb may aggravate the pain. The pain may last for days or weeks and the patient may be none the worse for it.

The shoulder may be involved in periarthritis (frozen shoulder) and becomes painful with the limitation of its movements. Severe pain in the arm may result from cervical Spondylosis.

Sometimes, these chest pains of non-cardiac origin and frozen shoulder occur after a heart attack. The patient may become unduly apprehensive, till he is informed by the physician that the pain is not cardiac in origin and does not presage another heart attack.

Is this knowledge sufficient for me to distinguish cardiac pain from non-cardiac pain?

I do not suggest that you try to diagnose the cause of your chest pain or palpitations yourself. That can be dangerous.

But I do want to inform you that there are chest pains arising not from the heart but from other structures such as joints, muscles and ligaments. Even though the pain caused by these structures is sometimes very severe, it is not of great consequence, whereas the heart pain, howsoever mild, will have to be taken seriously and treated properly.

Doctor, how do you distinguish these non-cardiac symptoms from true cardiac disease?

An experienced physician will be able to distinguish between cardiac pain and non-cardiac pain, as well as between palpitations caused by heart disease and functional consciousness of heart action. A careful study of the history of the illness and physical examination coupled with a routine ECG is usually all that may be necessary, but in some cases, further observation and investigations may become necessary to arrive at a proper diagnosis.

21

Related Disorders

Arterial obstruction and occlusion by fatty deposits (atheroma) are not confined to the coronary arteries. This is a general disease of the arteries. It occurs in the aorta and its larger branches, especially those of the brain and the lower limbs. By the age of 60, most people can be presumed to have atheromatous lesions spread over their arterial tree. Such lesions may be profound in those who have been indulging in an unhealthy life-style marked by factors such as excessive smoking, lack of physical activity, obesity, hypertension and uncontrolled diabetes.

Why to you want to discuss the aforementioned disorders in a book on heart attacks?

These related disorders are mentioned here for three reasons. First, a patient of ischaemic heart disease may, in addition, exhibit symptoms related to the brain. It is not uncommon for a patient to have repeated transient ischaemic attacks of the brain and then have a heart attack or hemiplegia. Secondly, vascular surgery is making rapid progress and it is becoming increasingly feasible to replace diseased arteries, where accessible, with artificial ones. Thirdly, we must examine how much we stand to make additional gains by taking precautions against coronary artery disease.

Do these lesions also create as many problems as the coronary artery lesions?

The lesions in the aorta may remain completely symptomless unless they produce obstructions at critical points like the bifurcation of the aorta. The lesions in the legs are much less likely to create problems than the coronary artery lesions. The lesions in the arteries of the brain also may remain symptomless until and unless clotting of blood on a lesion or a spasm of the artery produces stoppage of the blood flow. These lesions can also lead to problems if the blood pressure suddenly falls to very low levels, say, due to a heart attack or after taking an excessively large dose of antihypertensive drugs. In such situations, the blood flow through the already partially obstructed arteries may come to a standstill and cause thrombosis (clot) and produce infarction of the brain. After the heart, the brain is the next most frequently affected organ.

How does the blockage of the artery of the leg manifest itself?

The atheroma of the artery of the leg may be symptomless, or may cause ischaemic pain in the calf muscle while walking, which can be relieved by rest. This is called 'intermittent claudication'. Clotting of blood may sometimes occur in the diseased artery, blocking the artery completely and cutting off the blood supply to the part of the limb below the blockage. This results in gangrene of the leg.

What are the symptoms produced by blockage higher up at the bifurcation of the aorta?

Blockage at this level causes claudication to occur in the buttocks and thigh along with importence (in males).

What happens when the arteries leading to the brain are involved?

The occlusions occurring in the arteries of the brain may cause symptoms related to that organ. They may cause temporary reversible ischaemia of the brain or may result in infarction of the brain tissue, i.e., stroke. The symptoms would depend upon the specific area of the brain that suffers ischaemia or infarction, as different areas of the brain control different functions of the body. The patient may, therefore, suffer from various types of paralyses, blindness, disturbances of the intellect, memory or speech, etc. If the affliction is due to temporary ischaemia, complete recovery may occur in a few hours. The attacks are called 'transient ischaemic attacks' (TIA). If infarction, i.e., death of the brain tissue, has occurred, the damage is permanent and is called a 'stroke'.

What about the risk factors for the brain and the occurrence of peripheral arterial disease?

Despite the strong association between coronary atheroma and cerebral (brain) atheroma, the risk factors relating to the latter are not so clearly understood as those of the former. However, hypertension is a factor which seems common to both. Smoking is as much a factor in the causation of peripheral arterial disease of the legs as of the heart. The role of other factors, such as diabetes, obesity and high blood cholesterol, in the causation of cerebral arterial disease is not yet fully defined. However, on the basis of the present state of knowledge, all precautions to be observed for heart diseases should be considered useful to prevent cerebral and peripheral arterial diseases.

22

Epilogue

By now, you must have obtained a fairly good idea about ischaemic heart disease, i.e., angina pectoris and heart attacks; how these conditions are investigated, diagnosed and treated by doctors. You have learnt that IHD is caused by the clogging of the arteries of the heart by fatty deposits, thereby obstructing the flow of blood in these arteries. The prevention of heart disease lies in preventing the clogging of these arteries. Some of the factors responsible for heart attacks cannot be helped. For instance, you cannot help aging nor can you help being a male, if you are one, nor can you have any choice over your parentage and heredity. But you can do a lot to control and possibly eliminate risk factors such as cigarette smoking, consumption of animal fats, obesity, stress, high blood pressure, diabetes and excess of alcohol. There is the good news for the cigarette smokers. If they stop smoking cigarettes, their susceptibility to heart attacks drops down to about the same level as that of a non-smoker within a year or two. So, better stop smoking forthwith. Reduce your weight to the ideal level. Cut down animal fats and start using vegetable oils as a cooking medium. Avoid fried food totally. Cut down on red meat, if you are a non-vegetarian and go in for fish. A vegetarian diet with fresh vegetables and fruits would prove highly beneficial. Perform exercise regularly, compatible with your age and physical capacity. Avoid stress, loss of temper and working against time. Stop looking at your watch too often, and make yourself a little free from avoidable tension. Maintain a steady moderate pace of work. Cultivate methods of relaxation like meditation. Slow down your pace of life as age advances, yet remaining active till the end. Reduce alcohol intake. If you have high blood pressure or diabetes, keep them under control with the guidance of your doctor. Remember that these diseases last lifelong and so will be their management.

Above all LIVE YOUR AGE.

If a heart attack does occur, you have learnt how to recognize the symptoms or at least suspect them. I would again stress that the severity of pain is no criterion of the severity of the attack. Many attacks may occur without much pain or even with no pain at all, simply with sudden excessiveweakness and cold sweat. They need as much care as attacks accompanied by pain.

If you suffer from anginal pain, consult your doctor immediately, so that he can treat you for this condition. With a view to preventing major catastrophes from occurring, the precautions already outlined should be strictly followed.

If you have in you any evidence of IHD or have risk factors for the heart, don't forget your daily dose of aspirin.

You must prepare yourself to treat cardiac arrest. Practise regularly the technique of external cardiac massage and perfect it. Teach it to everyone around you at home and place of work, your friends, in fact any one you come across. You never know who will need it and when. You might need the massage yourself. Remember you have only $3^1/_2$ minutes to save the person who has suffered a cardiac arrest. No doctor can possibly reach the victim in such a short time. You have to act as the doctor at that time. Remember the thump on the chest and the cardiac massage are far more important than haphazardly running to locate a telephone or searching for a doctor. Somebody else in the vicinity should be doing that job, whom you may shout for help.

If you save even one life, you would have achieved a great deal.

I hope you have enjoyed reading the book. Armed with this knowledge and by putting it into pratice, I hope you will live healthy to a ripe old age and also assist others in achieving this objective.

Appendix 1

Hints on Food

1. Food for the Obese

(a) *Consume Freely:*

- Beans, cabbage, cauliflower, carrots, cucumber, lettuce, mushrooms, onions, pumpkin, radish, spinach, turnip, brinjal, ladies' finger, *tinda,* and *gheea* (different types of gourds).
- Fruits (without added sugar): lemon, oranges, malta, melons, *keenu* (an orange like fruit), strawberries, raspberries, grape-fruit, *mosammi.*
- Tea or coffee without sugar, soda water, lemon juice, tomato juice, diabetic fruit squash, clear unthickened soup, soup made of chicken or beef cubes.
- Artificial sweetening agents (such as saccharine), salt and pepper, vinegar, mustard, herbs, *masalas,* flavourings and colourings.

(b) *Avoid consuming:*

- Sugar, *gur* (jaggery) and glucose.
- Sweets, toffees, chocolates, chocolate biscuits, cream biscuits, and similar items.

- *Halwai* sweets: *jalebi, gulab jamun, rasgullas, ras-malai, burfi, peda,* and *balushahi.*
- Sweet dishes: *halwa,* custard, cornflour, *firni* and puddings.
- Jams, marmalades and honey.
- Tinned fruits and *murabbas.*
- Dried fruits: dates, figs, apricots and *sultanas (kishmish).*
- Fruits (very sweet): mangoes and grapes.
- Cakes, buns and pastries.
- Cereals: rice, spaghetti and macaroni.
- Breakfast cereals, porridge.
- Beverages such as Cocoa, Boost, Bournvita and Horlicks.
- Ice-creams, fresh cream, fruit cream.
- Condensed milk.
- Nuts.
- Salad cream, salad dressing, mayonnaise.
- Thickened sauces.
- Sweet pickles and chutneys.
- Thickened soups and gravies.
- Alcoholic drinks: beer, wines, sherry, spirits.
- Sweetened fruit juices, fruit squash.
- Cola drinks and other sweet fizzy drinks.
- Sausages.
- Butter, *malai,* egg yolk, *ghee,* vegetable oil (except the minimum amount necessary for cooking).
- All fried foods like *parathas, samosa,* and *pakoras.*

Cook the food any way you like—boiling, grilling, steaming or baking, but do not fry in *ghee* or oil.

(c) *All other foodstuffs not mentioned in either of the above two categories should be taken in moderation.*

2. Food for the Diabetic

(a) *Avoid altogether:*

- Sugar, glucose and *gur* (jaggery).
- Jams, marmalade and *murabbas.*
- Syrups, *sherbet* and honey.
- Tinned fruits.
- Sweets like toffees and chocolates and *halwai* sweets.
- Sweet biscuits, chocolate biscuits and cream biscuits.
- Cola, lemonade and other fizzy drinks, glucose drinks.
- Sweetened milk preparations and condensed milk.
- Cakes, pastries, pies, puddings and thick sauces.
- Alcoholic drinks: beer, wines, spirits.

(b) *Consume in moderation:*

- *Chapattis.*
- Bread, white or brown.
- Biscuits (not sweet).
- Breakfast cereals and porridge.
- All fresh and dried fruits.
- Macaroni, spaghetti, custard, cornflour.
- Thick soups.
- Diabetic foods.
- Milk (low fat) and its products.
- Pulses (*dals*).
- Eggs.
- Red meats.
- Potatoes, peas and baked beans.

(c) *Eat as much as you like:*

- All white meats and fish.
- Clear soups.
- Meat extracts.
- Tomato juice, lemon juice and orange juice.

- Tea or coffee (without sugar).
- Fresh vegetables: cauliflower, spinach, turnip, brinjals, ladies' finger, *tinda, gheea,* French beans, onions, mushrooms, lettuce, cucumber, spring onions, radish, *karela* (bitter gourd).
- Spices and herbs, salt, pepper and mustard.
- Artificial sweetening agents such as saccharine.

For obese or overweight diabetics, all fats (animal or vegetable) should be restricted and fried foods in all forms should be banned.

3. Low Cholesterol Food

The food items should be high in polyunsaturated fat content and low in saturated fats and cholesterol.

(a) *Use:*

- Polyunsaturated oil; e.g., sunflower oil, safflower oil, soyabean or corn oil, instead of *ghee* or other animal fats as a cooking medium.

(b) *Avoid:*

- Butter.
- Hydrogenated margarine.
- All animal fats: *ghee,* lard, suet.
- Cakes, biscuits and pastries made with the above ingredients.
- *Halwai* sweets made from animal fats.
- Fatty meats and organ meats (brain, liver, kidney).
- Whole milk and cream.
- Chocolates, ice-cream and fruit-cream.
- Cheese.
- Coconut and coconut oil.
- Eggs.
- Shell fish.
- All fried foods, except those fried in unsaturated oil.

Appendix 2

Desirable Body Weights

(minimum clothing; without shoes)

Height		Men	Women
ft. in	cm	kg	kg
4.10	148	–	48-51
4.11	150	–	49-52
5.00	153	–	51-54
5.01	156	–	52-55
5.02	158	56-60	53-57
5.03	161	58-62	54-58
5.04	163	59-64	56-60
5.05	166	61-65	58-61
5.06	168	62-67	59-64
5.07	171	64-69	61-65
5.08	173	66-71	62-67
5.09	176	68-73	64-69

Contd...

Height		Men	Women
ft. in	cm	kg	kg
5.10	178	69-74	66-70
5.11	181	71-76	67-72
6.00	184	73-79	69-74
6.01	186	75-81	–
6.02	189	78-84	–
6.03	191	80-86	–

SIMPLIFIED FORMULA FOR MAXIMUM DESIRABLE BODY WEIGHT

Men	5 feet	55 kg
Women	5 feet	52 kg

Add 2 kg per extra inch of height.

Glossary

ANGINA: Heart pain of short duration, usually located in the front of the chest.

ANGIOGRAPHY: X-ray of the blood vessels after injection of radio-opaque substance.

ANEURYSM: Localized abnormal dilation of an artery, aorta or the heart.

ANEURYSMECTOMY: Surgical removal of the sac of aneurysm.

ANGIOPLASTY: Plastic surgery performed on a blood vessel.

AORTA: The largest artery of the body into which the heart pumps the blood and which distributes this blood to the whole body through its numerous branches.

ARTERY: A tube-like structure that carries blood from the heart to the tissues.

ATHEROMA: A plaque of fatty deposit in the wall of an artery.

ATRIUM: A chamber of the heart which receives the blood from the body (right) or from the lungs (left).

BICYCLE ERGOMETERY: A stationary cycle used in determining the amount of work performed by the rider.

BLOOD VESSELS: The tubes that carry blood, i.e., arteries and veins.

CARDIAC ARREST: Sudden stoppage of the heart beat.

CONTRAST MEDIUM: Radio-opaque substance used for X-ray work, including angiography.

CORONARY BYPASS: A shunt established surgically which permits blood to travel from the aorta to a branch of the coronary artery at a point past an obstruction, bypassing the latter.

ECHOCARDIOGRAPHY: A non-invasive diagnostic method that uses ultrasound waves to visualise internal structures of the heart.

EMBOLISM: Obstruction of a blood vessel by a blood clot (embolus) brought from a thrombus in a distant blood vessel.

HYPERTENSION: High blood pressure.

ICCU: Intensive coronary care unit.

IHD or ISCHAEMIC HEART DISEASE or CORONARY HEART DISEASE: Narrowing and thus causing obstruction of the coronary artery due to atheroma, which is sufficient to prevent adequate blood supply to the heart muscle, causing angina and heart attack.

INFARCT: An area of necrosed (dead) tissue following cessation of blood supply to it.

ISCHAEMIA: (pronounced *is-kee-mia*): Inadequate flow of blood to a part caused by obstruction to its blood supply.

LIPID: Fat.

LUMEN: Bore of a blood vessel.

MYOCARDIAL INFARCTION: Death of a part of the heart muscle following cessation of blood supply to it; acute heart attack.

NECROSIS: Area of dead tissue surrounded by a healthy area.

RESUSCITATION: Revival after apparent death.

SCINTISCAN: Use of scintiphotography to produce a map of scintillations produced when a radioactive substance is introduced into the body. The intensity of the record indicates the differential accumulation of the radioactive substance in various parts of the body.

THROMBOSIS: Formation of a blood clot (thrombus) within a blood vessel.

TISSUE: A collection of similar cells which act together in the performance of a particular function; e.g., muscle, nerve.

VEIN: A tube that carries blood from the tissues back to the heart.

VENTRICLE: A chamber of the heart which pumps blood into the aorta (left) or into the lungs (right).

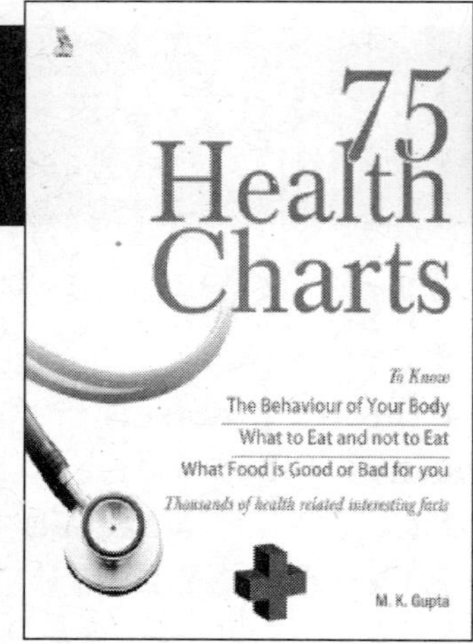

75 Health Charts

—M. K. Gupta

As any health-conscious person knows, health is truly wealth. Yet, simply harbouring good intentions does not ensure good health for anyone. Beginning in infancy and right up to our twilight years, a conscious attempt has to be made to lead a healthy lifestyle. In the formative years, our parents make this effort on our behalf. But as we enter the teens and take control of our own destinies, how well informed we are on health-related issues makes all the difference between physical well-being and ill health.

This book ensures you have all the facts, figures and data at your fingertips to promote proper health and nutrition in order to prevent disease.

In this book you will find: height and weight charts, blood pressure and pulse rate charts, calorie charts, fat and cholesterol charts, vitamin and mineral charts, balanced diet charts, pollution health hazard charts, infectious diseases and immunisation charts, healthy heart and stress charts... not to mention other relevant charts, tables and data.

So, if health has always been your problem, this book is just what the doctor ordered. And if health has been your forte, this book is exactly what the doctor would recommend to maintain you in the pink of your health. Either way, *75 Health Charts* is a must-read for all people.

Big Size • Pages: 144
Price: Rs. 120/- • Postage: Rs. 25/-

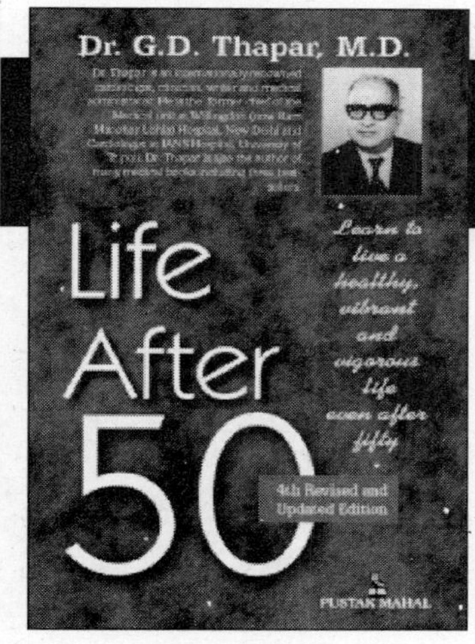

Life After Fifty

—Dr. G.D. Thapar, M.D.

This authoritatively written book focuses on the second innings of your life. It deals exhaustively with every facet of life which is linked with our natural process of ageing and explains the ability of the body which is really great, provided it is put to judicious and optimal use.

Written in a simple language, the author reveals that life is a series of adaptations. Healthy habits based on common sense principles and the readiness to act, if and when problem arises, enables one to lead a vigorous life during the advanced years. It helps you to—

- Find an appropriate occupation for the elderly.
- Be happy, though retired.
- Cope with stress.
- Physically fit and mentally active.

Aim for advanced years free from chronic diseases and depression, for a life full of eternal youth and vigour.

Demy Size • Pages: 192
Price: Rs. 150/- • Postage: Rs. 25/-

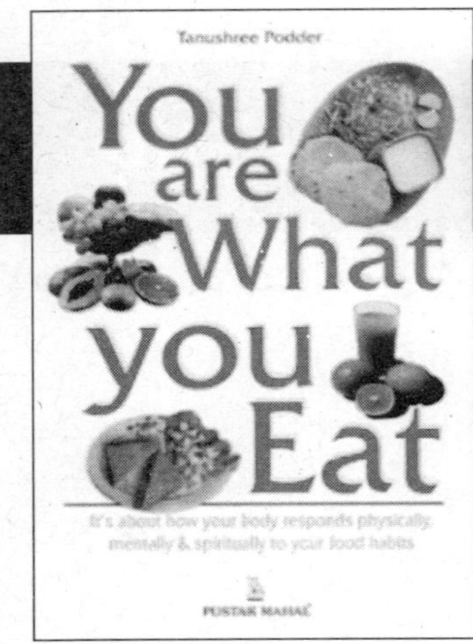

You are What you Eat

—Tanushree Podder

It's about how your body responds physically, mentally & spiritually to your food habits

Did you know that food could heal, cure, elevate moods, improve memory, make the brain sharper, provide us with potent energy and fill us with vigour?

Food has been discovered to be the greatest natural pharmacy that is available to human beings. The right food can help us perform to our peak capacity while the wrong food can lead us towards disease and ill health.

The ordinary cabbage and cauliflower could ward off the possibility of cancer, tomatoes can effectively take care of free radicals in today's environment and carrots can provide you with the essential beta-carotene to fight off many diseases. It is surprising how effectively food can alleviate most of our common ailments.

The mysteries of the power of food and the secrets of food elements have been unravelled so that you can use food for other benefits rather than just appeasing hunger.

Demy Size • Pages: 184
Price: Rs. 96/- • Postage: Rs. 25/-

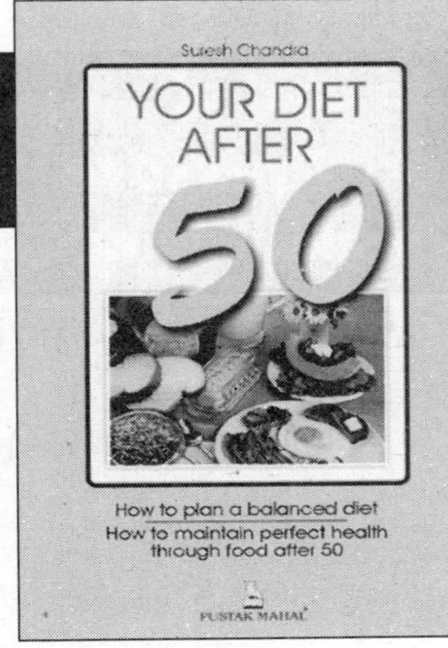

Your Diet After 50

—Suresh Chandra

Your life is filled with choices. Everyday you make choices related to clothes, shoes and sometimes marriage proposals and jobs, for your sons and daughters, if not for yourself. Some seem trivial, while others are important. But apart from these, there is one choice which can have a major impact on your health and your life.

This book is about the choice of food—food that is nutritious and health giving. Within its pages, you will find reliable nutritional information and sound advice, based on scientific evidence. It offers you practical ways to eat healthy in almost any situation and at every phase of life, particularly after 50. And it encourages you to enjoy the pleasures of food but, at the same time, promote your health and well-being. After all, taste is the number one reason why most people choose one food over the another. Most important, the flexible guidelines help you choose nutritious, flavourful foods to match your own needs, preferences and lifestyle, even as your life enters the third phase.

Demy Size • Pages: 152
Price: Rs. 96/- • Postage: Rs. 25/-

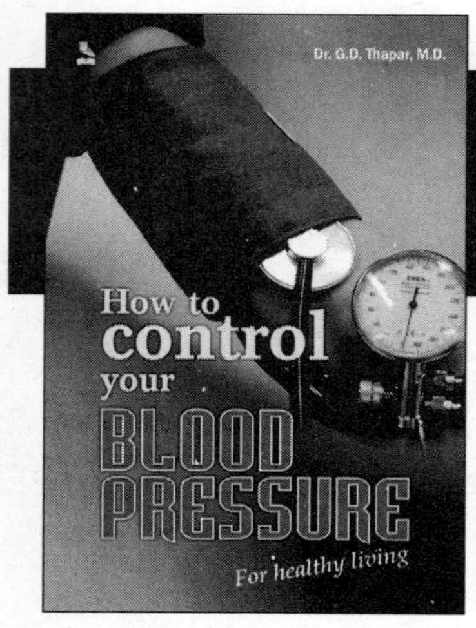

How to control your
Blood Pressure
For healthy living

—Dr. G.D. Thapar, M.D.

Hypertension has been termed as a 'Silent Killer', because it produces few symptoms but continues doing its damage. Symptoms arise from its complications, most of which are serious conditions like heart attacks and strokes.

Consequently, everybody needs to possess some basic, relevant and accurate information and facts about this killer disease to prevent it in the first instance and control it, if necessary.

The book helps you in identifying the causes and development of adverse effects of Hypertension. It also gives information on major hypertension-related diseases and gives physiological and other measures for controlling hypertension and preventing its complications. Many of the queries arising in the minds of the readers are answered in the book.

Demy Size • Pages: 126
Price: Rs. 120/- • Postage: Rs. 25/-

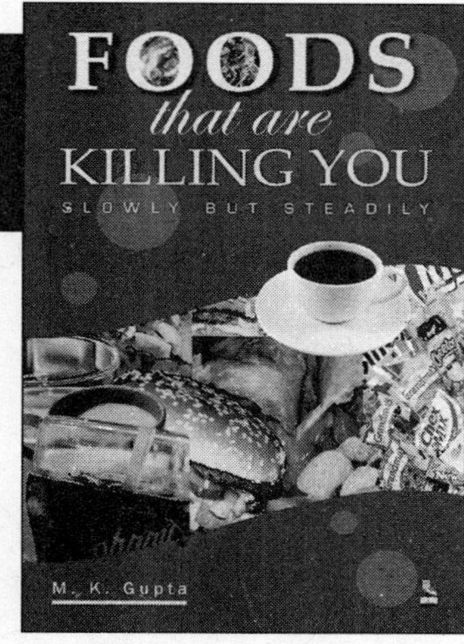

Foods that are Killing You

—M. K. Gupta

It is truly said: *You are what you eat.* Although most of us have heard this axiom, we don't bother to give it a second thought. That is why, white sugar, table salt, fatty and acidic foods and the wrong food combinations, besides other pesticide-laden foods, are part of our everyday menu.

Foods that are Killing You seeks to increase awareness among readers about wrong eating habits that end up destroying our health and silently killing us. The book also highlights the dangers of consuming coffee, tea, alcohol and milk – yes, milk!

The harmful effects of all these foods are explained in explicit terms. Proper scientific understanding of the side effects of such harmful foods can ensure that we eliminate or control the consumption of foodstuffs containing excess pesticides and cholesterol, leading to enhanced well-being and better health. This book is a must in every home, because health is truly wealth.

Demy Size • Pages: 160
Price: Rs. 100/- • Postage: Rs. 25/-